The Art of Becoming
a Nurse Healer

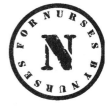

The Art of Becoming
a Nurse Healer

by Beverly A. Hall RN, PhD, FAAN

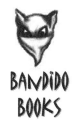

BANDIDO
BOOKS

Includes references. Orlando, Florida 2005

ISBN 1-929693-49-4

Cover art direction by David Morales
Cover picture "Strange Colors" by Harald Wittmaack
Printed in the United States of America

To learn more about similar titles in the *For Nurses by Nurses Series* and to keep abreast of our latest offerings for nursing professionals, please visit us at *www.bandidobooks.com* or contact us via email at *publish@bandidobooks.com* or by postal service at:

Bandido Books
9806 Heaton Court
Orlando, FL 32817

Nursing at Clinical Speed!

For order information call our toll-free hotline at 1.877.817.6824
PIN 1174

About the Author

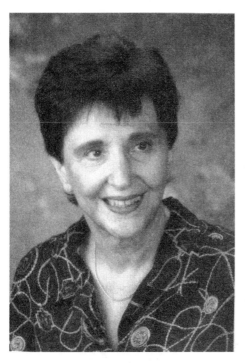

Beverly Hall, PhD, RN, FAAN is Professor Emeritus, University of Texas at Austin, School of Nursing. Previously, she was Professor and Chair of the Department of Mental Health, Community, and Administrative Nursing, University of California San Francisco. Dr. Hall is a psychiatric nurse and a medical sociologist. She has conducted research on living with HIV and developed community programs for HIV care. She has worked with patients at the end stage of life. Her counseling of people with serious life threatening illnesses culminated in a book, *Surviving and Thriving After a Life Threatening Diagnosis* (2004). She has written more than 65 articles and books in the area of health, health promotion, and healing, and for years has presented university classes, professional and public lectures, and workshops on various topics of theory, research, health, and patient care. She now lives in Baltimore, Maryland. She invites your comments on this book at *bevhall@mail.utexas.edu*

Acknowledgements

I owe a real debt of gratitude to the thousands of students and patients who have been part of my life for more than 30 years and through their examples have taught me to be a healing nurse. I owe special appreciation to Janet Allan, my friend and companion. She read and evaluated every word of this book and provided astute scrutiny in gentle way that sent me back to the drawing board with renewed insight. I would like to acknowledge the support of Arizona friends, Jim Alsip and Laura Isenstein, who encouraged me through the production of several publications and used their influence as librarians to guide me toward crucial resources. I owe more than I can say to Peggy Chinn whose powerful ideas over the years have enhanced the analytic ability of both my right and my left brain.

Thank you to the 5 reviewers who gave generously of their time to provide so many well thought out ideas, suggestions, and questions. By your critique you raised the quality and usefulness of the book enormously. Thanks to my neighbor Brett Pekens for enlightening me on how to construct a boat that could sail beyond the sunset. Living near the harbor in Baltimore afforded an inspiration from the water and brought me in contact with sailors who will one day attempt to cruise beyond the sunset, if for no other reason, just to see what is behind there.

My deepest thanks to Martin Schiavenato, Editor-in-Chief, Bandido Books for his support and his encouragement to pursue a style of writing that is readable and informal. This personal approach permitted me to reach out to readers in the same welcoming way that I advocate that nurses reach out to patients.

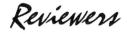
Reviewers

Marie-Annette Brown RN, PhD, FNP, FAAN
Professor, University of Washington, School of Nursing
Nurse Practitioner and Primary Care provider, Women's Health
Clinic, University Washington Medical Center.

Peggy L. Chinn RN, PhD, FAAN
Professor Emerita, University of Connecticut.

Pamela A. Minarik APRN BC, MS, FAAN
Professor and Director, Office of International Affairs,
Yale University School of Nursing, and
Psychiatric Consultation Liaison Clinical Nurse Specialist,
Yale-New Haven Hospital.

Sharon L. Moore RN, BA, M.Ed., PhD
Associate Professor,
Centre for Nursing and Health Studies,
Athabasca University.

Kristen M. Swanson RN, PhD, FAAN
Professor and Chairperson,
Family and Child Nursing,
University of Washington.

In memory of my parents

Lois Mae Hall
Leslie L. Hall

Any ability that I now have to be an imaginative and independent thinker I owe to the upbringing of my talented mother and father who always knew that I would set my sights well beyond the sunset.

Table of Contents

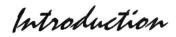

Building a Ship to Sail Beyond the Sunset

Come, my friend, 'tis not too late to see a newer world. Push off, and sitting well in order to smite the sounding furrows, for my purpose holds to sail beyond the sunset.
-Tennyson

My last 5 years as a Professor of Nursing at the University of Texas at Austin, I taught two theory courses to hundreds of master's degree students, primarily those preparing to be nurse practitioners. These highly successful courses were focused on learning the theoretical and practical foundations of nursing practice. Several years after the course was over I was still hearing from some of these students as they expressed their gratitude and described the difference it made in their ability to be good nurses and to derive satisfaction from their practice.

The course in its own way was a miracle. That first class of students grudgingly dragged themselves to my class, positive that the content would consist of the same dry "nursing theory" that had been the great soporific they had experienced as undergraduates. At some early point in the semester, for about the third of the class, a switch turned on in the student's mind, as the class began to grasp the implications of something that felt different and at first inexplicable. As the semester wore on, new lights literally blazed in student's heads. A great many were amazed that the same nursing phenomena that they had been observing for years had been transformed before their eyes into something unique and powerful. I had always felt that I was a good teacher, but the reviews that I got for those courses far exceeded anything I had ever before achieved, and in subsequent semesters, I refined the content and improved my methods of teaching it. A major factor in its success was that the lectures formed a pattern that promoted a form of care that was more advanced technologically and spiritually than anything they had encountered before. What I will present in the following pages draws heavily from that experience. My aim is to foreground a form of nurse healing that you will find so useful that you will wonder how you ever practiced the old way.

I will begin here as I asked these students to begin. Think back over your years in practice, about a moment when you really felt like a nurse – when you became aware of incredible strength in your ability to achieve an outcome that was effective for a patient. I will bet that it was a time when you stopped whatever else you were doing in order to give the most of your skill and knowledge that you could give at that moment. Or perhaps it was when you felt such empathy and concern for another person that you took a minute to be fully there. Or maybe it was after you left the patient, and realized with certainty and a glow of self-admiration that you had displayed the strength to get through a tough situation with grace and dignity.

Unfortunately these moments are rare in nursing, not just today – they always have been, and there are many reasons why this is so. Nursing schools have routinely taught theories about empathy while at the same time rewarding objectivity. "Don't get too involved," you are warned. "It saps your ability to do your job." For another, nurses have busy lives and we all have our own problems that we bring to work that to a large extent shape our responses to others. Nobody tells us how to practice in a way that helps us resolve our own problems as we are dealing with those of the patients. Most importantly, we lack support from professional colleagues – the collaboration and backing that would help us go beyond delivering routine care. Moreover, it goes without saying that even routine care is now so complex that it takes enough energy and knowledge without feeling that one has to add on other less tangible factors into the busy life of a nurse. And finally, a major reason why nurses do not incorporate healing into their nursing practice is that they simply do not know what it is. Nor do they know how to do it, how to sustain it, or how to work it into their daily routine of patient care.

What is healing in nursing, or nursing care that is beyond routine? In a book that has the words "Nurse Healer" in the title, it might be expected that I will say some touchy-feely thing, or suggest ways to provide emotional support, or discuss alternative healing methods, but none of this is the case. Healing derives from a sense of hope, a view that in every single instance, there is always something we can do to alleviate suffering, and that we own the responsibility to think through the alternatives. Therefore, as Quinn[1] helps us to realize, the healing model is always optimistic because nurses can always heal even when patients cannot be cured. Healing develops out of learning how to be in right relation with self and others. It is based on intentionality, compassion, and the focused attention of the nurse toward the patient. Patients who cannot be cured of their disease can be healed because healing, derived from the Greek word *haelen*, means to make whole.[1] A state of wholeness exists as entirely separate from the patient's disease. We can be as whole in sickness as we are in health.

Making whole is based upon a sense of spirituality. Most of the patients who come under our care have a critical disease that is frightening and for some will end in serious disability or death. Medical techniques can be supportive and palliative, but often cannot reverse this inevitable progression. Yet when nurses strive to make the critically ill patient whole, this "thing that we do" puts nurses in a wonderful position to be of service to patients. Seizing the many opportunities to be in service to patients is not only your great gift to patients, it will turn out to be a great gift to you.

My experiences in healing have made me ever more aware of my own reasons for being a nurse. While counseling patients with the serious, life-threatening diagnoses of cancer and HIV, and caring for patients dying in a hospice, I began to understand that my purpose in being there was to experience life fully through attending to the challenges set forth by their suffering and their accruing perceptions derived from living in pain and fear. I learned to regard my patients as teachers because of their developing insight about the end of life, and their fortitude in the ways they confronted something that I was struggling with, but had yet to experience.

At first, I marveled at their grit and tranquility in the face of death. Later, as I grew in maturity, I marveled at my own courage that allowed me to connect with them in a journey that was entirely without signposts. Through my investments in them, I learned that I was actually supposed to take on all the happiness and the pain that are products of being human, not to race with ears covered and eyes blindfolded through the bad parts while hoping for a better day tomorrow. I learned to dwell with them through their dying, not in a detached, cowardly way, but in a way that allowed me to participate fully in the process. I learned that while anyone can enjoy living during times of peak enjoyment, it is also possible to take satisfaction in life from suffering. I discovered that my personal spiritual path involved understanding my commitments to self and others, and I accepted that what was happening at any moment was never some awful, terrible thing, but rather exactly what was supposed to be happening. It almost goes without mentioning that the growth that I experienced as a nurse followed me into my personal life, allowing me to rise above my fear of dying and to connect with others in a way that permitted an enriched commitment to living.

We become nurse healers when we follow a personal and spiritual path that helps us strive to be the very best we can.[2] It is giving as much as you have to give in the performance of any nursing task, whether technical, physical, or emotionally supportive.[3] Being a healer further directs us as nurses to use whatever means are at our disposal to advocate for our patients and to engage in actions that are in our patient's best interest. It involves using nursing knowledge to make people as comfortable as they can be. It means using intellectual reasoning to solve the seemingly unsolvable problems that sick and frightened patients present every day – intractable pain, infection, ravishes of internal disease, signs of giving up on themselves, being uncooperative with care, not engaging with treatment – while looking beyond the obvious indicators, and sensing the underlying drama that is taking place in the patient's world. It means being in touch with yourself, with your reactions, as you respond to the diverse and sometimes difficult personalities that any nurse meets every day. To sum it up, nurse healing arises out of making good judgments, being attentive and responsible, and caring about what happens.

The remaining chapters in this book will show that healing in nursing is not all that difficult to learn, and that the gains for both patient and nurse are enormous. In healing, you always get two for one – anytime you work at caring for another, you are caring for yourself as well. But at the outset, if you are wondering why any nurse should bother about doing nursing that goes beyond the routine – going beyond what is required by orders and care plans - I ask you to engage in one simple exercise that involves remembering a time when one of your close friends or family was in the hospital. Did you trust the nursing personnel enough to relax in the certainty that they would provide the model of care you wanted for your family or friend? As an insider you know how chaotic the system is in which nurses practice, and how unconcerned many exhausted and busy nurses appear at times when regarding the welfare of their patients. Did you have full assurance that your family member would receive the top care that is your highest standard for them?

When you look back on experiences you have had with your family in health care, I expect you will realize that what separates barely adequate care from excellent care is often something that is very simple and easy to deliver if someone would just take a second to work with the patient. Here are two examples of my own, and I have found that every nurse has dozens of stories like these.

My friend, Susan was in the hospital after surgery. They removed her urinary catheter the morning she was supposed to be discharged. The LPN informed us that she would not be discharged until she voided, and then left the room. I escorted a wobbly and sleepy Susan to the bathroom 3 times where she sat, but could not urinate. After an hour or so went by, I went to the desk and reported to the LPN that she still could not void. She confirmed that we had to keep trying because until she voided she could not leave. I knew about some simple things like running water, but as a psychiatric nurse, it was beyond my expertise to figure this out. So after more than 2 hours, I went looking for help and saw a sign on a door that said, DEBORAH BROWN, CLINICAL NURSE SPECIALIST. I walked into Ms. Brown's office and said, "Please, could you help us," and I told her what the problem was. She came back to Susan's room with me and worked diligently with us for a short time, trying different things until finally, Susan urinated and was able to be discharged. I thanked Ms. Brown profusely and complemented her on the way that she worked this through. I could tell that she was proud of her efforts on our behalf, despite the fact that this was not a terribly difficult problem for someone with her training. But had I not sought her out, not a soul would have come to help who was knowledgeable and willing to offer the expertise it took to solve the problem.

The second example concerns my own mother who was dying from cancer of the pancreas and in intractable pain. When I came back to the hospital after work, to spend the night with her, she was in horrible pain and I learned that she had been vomiting all day. The vomiting was increasing her pain immensely. I could hardly stand to see my mother in that condition. I found out that they had tried anti-nausea medication, so I asked the nurse if she would get an order for another type of anti-nausea drug. This medication did not alleviate the problems either, so I asked the nurse what else could be the cause, since this had come on so suddenly. The nurse could not think of a thing. So I asked her to look to see if any new medications had been ordered that might cause nausea, and we discovered that the resident had changed the pain medication the previous evening to try to get her more relief. I asked her to call the physician to see if we could restore the former pain medications, as it seemed obvious that an allergic response could be the culprit. After the order for the old pain medication was reinstated my mother's vomiting stopped and she was able to sleep for the first time in 24 hours.

In both examples, hospital nurses had been practicing a form of "routine nursing" that had involved following orders. In Susan's case, I forced Ms. Brown to be a good nurse, and when I did she was happy with the outcome of her care and proud of her nursing skills. In the second case, I led the nurse through a process of simple problem solving that she could have done easily without my help if she had been engaged and thoughtful. Don't get me wrong, the nurse caring for my mother was quite concerned about the vomiting, but she did not put her mind toward taking the next step that would transport her beyond her routine care. She did not engage with the patient or the situation. Engaging with the patient and the circumstances facing the patient while initiating steps to solve the problem, is at the heart of nurse healing.

Compellingly, Mother Theresa said that she could continue her work in the face of so much discouragement and difficulty because she was in a love relationship with everyone she met. This love was permitted because she saw the face of Christ in each person for whom she cared. My message here is not religious, so it is enough for me to believe that each nurse could be a nurse healer if only he or she would begin by seeing the face of her or his family members in every patient.

But what does it take to practice in a new way? What skill and knowledge are needed to help us discover who we could be and how we can sail into worlds beyond the sunset? We start with determining what kind of boat we will build for the journey. I would like to help you erect a sturdy boat that will proceed steadily and surely toward a landing, not one to race quickly toward the sunset to see how fast we can get there. On our boat we will meander occasionally, when it suits us, in order to savor the voyage. As we sail, we will not only rely on our scientific navigation instruments, we will also learn the art of reading the tides, the wind, the weather, and the sounds of the water lapping the side of the boat to chart corrections in our course. I want to take all the time we need to select the materials for the keel and the hull, and to lovingly mold them into a well-built and robust exterior in which we can have pride and confidence. At the same time, we will think of our own well being for the long haul in building the internal space, the space that will house us on the trip, in a way that promotes comfort and ease for our extended voyage.

So, I will present the knowledge and clinical intervention techniques that I and other nurses have learned from our engagement with practice and teaching hold the keys to arriving at our objective of healing the patient and the nurse. Integrating new ideas into practice will come to you as you study the entire book and as you deal with the discussion exercises at the end of each chapter. In fact, these exercises are a vital part of learning. I learned from my experience in teaching that students gained tremendous insights when they discussed them with their peers in school and at work. I devoted at least 1/3 of each class to small group discussion, providing a time when students could actually see that they were in a process of theory-practice integration that would serve them well as clinicians. So you will gain the most out of this book if you discuss it with a group of nurses at work or at school in ways that provoke ideas about significant clinical issues. For students in a distance learning course or nurses reading this alone, you will gain a great deal of insight by pondering the discussion questions in personal self study. Some of you might be able to arrange for a group in your workplace to read each chapter with you. Or, you might form a chat room with other students taking courses over the internet.

Discussion and Exercises

1. Recall a time when you really felt like a nurse. Describe that situation to the group. Break down the reasons why you felt useful and productive.

2. Describe the end result of that intervention for you and for the patient.

3. Remember a time when you visited a seriously ill family member or friend in the hospital and felt that the care was not as good as you would have given. What would you have done differently?

Part 1

Knowledge Base for the Nurse Healer

> *Inspire me with love for my art and for thy creatures.*
> *In the sufferer let me see only the human being.*
> *- Physician's Oath of Maimonides*

Nurse healing is primarily an art. This art has its roots in beauty; ethics, principles, and values; personal experience and personal involvement; and theories from scientific research. Our healing art is experienced by the patient as caring in the midst of ordinary interaction - caring that can be communicated in a flash, just by a nurse's presence while doing technical tasks, problem solving, or patient teaching. In this section, I will lay down a working version of the knowledge base that every nurse draws upon - knowledge that sets nursing apart as a discipline and allows a caring presence to become activated as nurse healing. The knowledge that is applied to healing is learned as a part of formal education and is ingrained into practice through experience. I have attuned this information to the realities of nursing practice so that nurses can draw on it to improve care.

Chapter 1

The Importance of Identifying Our Nursing Knowledge Base

Ideas about nursing knowledge must be both practical and understandable from a clinical perspective. While it is important to study textbook concepts for nursing practice, they only come to life as they become ingrained into a repertoire of practice that is so natural that after a while it requires little conscious thought. As a teacher of theory about nurse healing, I would much rather teach experienced nurses than a novice nurse who has not vaulted the fiery hurdles of practice, a nursing practice that consistently turns up too many serious problems and too few solutions. Experienced nurses are more than ready to begin a process of learning that they hope will result in being able to acquire knowledge that will guide them in solving some of the persistent problems they confront.

As intelligent and observant nurses, a great deal of what we know about patient responses is sensed intuitively or discovered by the trial and error of experience when caring for patients in states of trauma and illness and when working to overcome obstacles. Nursing, like other helping professions is an art that like all other arts, including painting and music, uses scientific principles. This is true of medicine as well. In a recent article, Dr. Catherine D. DeAngelis, editor of *Journal of the American Medical Association*, asserted that if medicine were strictly science, you could teach it to a computer. She said, "The thing that makes a physician a physician, or a nurse a nurse, or a clinician a clinician, is the personal aspect – the aspect that has more to do with the art." [4 (8a)]

As a nurse artist and a human being, your own life events sharpen your perceptions of crucial dilemmas in health care. For example, we can understand hope because we ourselves have felt hopeful and have felt its loss. When theories achieve this level of intuitive knowledge in practice, a nurse can quickly and easily access them for application to care in numerous situations. But, they also become inexplicable, existing largely on a non-verbal level. So establishing dependable and consistent communication about good practice from nurse to nurse is a major reason for codifying and writing down nursing knowledge. If nursing derives only from experience of an individual nurse than it has to be discovered over and over again by every nurse coming up the ranks – a real time waster.

For example, my first couple of months after graduation, I was working the night shift in the surgical recovery room, trying to apply my book knowledge to practice. Needless to say this was before the era of sophisticated monitors that nurses depend upon now. I worked along side Mrs. Jones, a nurse in her mid-sixties who went from patient to patient so rapidly that I did not see how she could ever be making the same assessments that I made. Yet, when a patient was getting into trouble, Mrs. Jones would be right there on top of things, even before it became apparent there was a problem, and she was working through the problem before I had even diagnosed it. I would ask her, "How did you know the patient was getting into trouble?" She could never answer that question. She just knew. "Great," I thought, "I would like to know, as well, and I would like to learn before I am 65 years old."

So theories can enhance our practice by pinpointing factors that require observations and pointing to general and specific solutions to problems. They serve specific purposes of:

- Suggesting cause and effect by telling us which events come first. Did the patient's loss of family support precede the patient's anger or did the patient's anger result in a loss of family support?
- Guiding our observations toward what is crucial. We simply cannot look at everything at once. We need a systematic way to collect, observe and organize a large amount of clinical data.
- Helping us to interpret what we see. It would be useless to take a body temperature if we lacked ideas about how the finding would be an indicator of health and disease.
- Moving us from seeing isolated facts to a more coherent way of thinking that helps us determine the significance of large numbers of facts, such as we find in a history or physical examination.

Discussion and Exercises

1. Describe a situation in detail in which a patient presented a problem that needed your attention.

   a. Identify all the factors that you think may be causing the problem. If possible, include the patient's own assessment of the cause.

   b. Identify which of these factors can be changed by nursing intervention.

2. When forming your way of intervening, identify where you think these practices came from. For example, did they come from your own or other's practice, from your personal experience with illness, from a nursing theory or a theory from another field?

Chapter 11

Knowledge for Nurse Healing is Ordinary Knowledge

The principal purpose of nursing care is to promote health and well being. Consequently nursing frameworks for practice are quite a bit broader than medical frameworks that are focused upon diagnosis and cure of disease. Nursing's Social Policy Statement,[5] describes nurses as protecting, promoting, and optimizing health. Individual nurses may at times feel that it is enough to concentrate on the medical problem and the patient's medical treatment, but despite this perception, nurses in practice do use a broader set of ideas. Nursing frameworks allow a focus on:

- Health and illness instead of diagnosis
- The human spirit as well as the mind and body
- Experience rather than prescription

Nursing knowledge is concerned with the *person* with the health concern, the *nurse* providing care, and the *environment* in which care is provided and the home environment where the patient became ill and where the patient will recover. Nurses know that people do not get sick or well in isolation, but rather that illness is a product of a large number of interacting factors both internal and external. In interrelating these three factors, our concern is with nurse-patient interaction within the relationship in which care is provided and the circumstances under which interaction and healing take place. It is in the context of this relationship and what surrounds it that the patient will derive the will, the power and the knowledge for healing.

Finally nursing is concerned with *health*, the desired end state for the patient, a broader goal than just having one's disease cured. Absence of disease is a very narrow view of health. Health is also the way that one feels every day, the energy to live a productive life, an ability to meet stated goals, the optimism that we bring to a task, and the state of our minds and bodies to resist illness and prevent disease. All people, even ill people have the right to pursue a healthy life, full of joy and meaning. Fawcett[6] has called the four italicized factors above – patient, nurse, environment, and health – nursing's metaparadigm.

A metaparadigm is an umbrella model that covers all of nursing. All theory, practice and research flow from these four concepts and from their interactions with each other. Different theories emphasize different concepts within the metaparadigm. For example in much of Florence Nightingale's writing she stressed that health was a desired outcome that could be produced by improvements in the patient's environment. To accomplish her goal, her nurses labored successfully to clean and sanitize as many as possible of the noxious elements that would come in direct contact with patients or with the air they breathed, thus preventing death from infection. Amazingly, her work was carried out well before the advent of the germ theory.

The fact that nurses direct attention to those factors that make up the metaparadigm means that although nurses may work with a patient to provide care that will cure or ameliorate a medical diagnosis, our paramount concern, as was Nightingale's, is the health of the patient in the environment. Prevention of illness is also an important part of health and falls within the nurse's domain. Although prevention has been much neglected in our haste to find more powerful treatments to cure disease, nurses in community health nursing have led the way for the rest of us in developing prevention as the main part of their intervention. The following is an old public health story that I have transformed a bit to illustrate this point:

> A group of doctors and nurses are standing by a river and see a baby floating by. They run in to pull her out. Then to their astonishment, more babies come and then more. These heroic clinicians work tirelessly through many days and nights trying to save all the babies floating down the river. Finally, most of the nurses along with a few of the doctors pull out and start running away. "Wait," the others cry. "How can you leave when all these babies need to be saved?" One of the nurses informed them, "We are going upstream to see who is throwing them in."

As nurses, we embrace the cure model, but a good part of our knowledge for practice is located upstream where we go to prevent them from getting thrown in. Much of our teaching is geared, not to treatment of disease, but to care that will enhance medical treatment and counseling that results in improvement of the patient's health and resistance to current and future illness. Moreover, nursing's concern is broader than the organ system that is affected, as we turn our attention to the emotional, physical, and spiritual health of the whole patient in a way that may or may not include the primary disease that brought the patient to medical care.

Given the above focus, Taylor[7] concluded that nursing knowledge is manifested as ordinary activities that we do for people because we care about their entire welfare. Added to our ordinary persona is competence. Being capable and skilled in using our knowledge base is the pinnacle of nurse healing. Both the patient and the nurse are human beings living a life. Caring for patients is a humanistic activity. It is a time when nurses can be equal with patients in day-to-day encounters, never above the patient, never looking down with learned pronouncements. In providing an ordinary form of caring, nurses do not have to put on "bedside manners" or other professional shields and facades when giving care. The most sophisticated and well educated nurse healer gives care in the guise of an ordinary person, a role that involves total absorption in healing. There is no room for the detached scientist in this picture, because nursing care requires personal engagement and authenticity.

Discussion and Exercises

1. As a group, write a clinical narrative that describes a common nursing phenomenon or use one from your practice.

   Examples of phenomena: comfort, rest and sleep; emotions helping or hindering the will to live; decision-making; social issues, such as poverty, lack of support; consumption issues, such as diet, alcohol, drugs, smoking; or multiple physical complaints.

   Begin to form a plan of care for this phenomenon under the headings Person, Nurse, Environment, and Health. Pay particular attention to how your plan of care addresses these concepts - how you are defining them in your plan, and the importance of each concept to the outcome you are seeking.

2. Come up with 3 or 4 examples of how you as a nurse provided care that was ordinary but effective.

3. Ask the group to talk about a time when they stopped pulling someone out of the river and went upstream. Hints: Smoking cessation, selected teaching and rehabilitation.

Chapter III

Ways of Knowing: An Overview

So many aspects of our life experiences affect what we know personally and professionally, and how we interpret what we hear and see. As early as 1978, Carper[8] identified the four patterns of knowing that are well accepted by nurse theorists: empirics, ethics, aesthetics, and personal. These patterns, or ways of knowing, have been discussed by many authors in the nursing theory literature, but none have added as much as the crucial work by Chinn and Kramer[9] in their book, *Theory and Nursing: Integrated Knowledge Development.* I urge the reader to access the latest edition of this highly readable, but scholarly book to extend and deepen the lessons about nursing knowledge that I will present here. I will refer to this work frequently but will not cover the same ground as they did. Readers need to refer to that source to gain a full appreciation of patterns of knowing in nursing.

All the ways of knowing are enriched by our experiences as nurses in the care of patients, by our personal beliefs, and the values that we accept as right and wrong for ourselves and others. You are influenced by the morals that your parents taught when you were young, by your religious upbringing, and current religious and spiritual involvement. Surprisingly, a large amount of your knowledge and way of seeing the world is a product of the talents and skills that you have honed over a life time. For example, I acquired my musical ability as a child growing up in a musical family. The way I approached it then has opened me to other forms of creativity, as I learned to play most of the instruments that I played then by my own instruction, with some occasional help from my father. I played along with records and the radio, learning to play by ear and improvise. I learned to take liberty with written music or ignore it entirely. As a result I have a great deal of confidence in using my own creativity to bring into being a satisfying outcome. When I am problem-solving a nursing dilemma in this creative way it promotes in me a sense of adventure – a glorious experience in improvising. When it comes to formulating nursing practice and theory development, I neither expect nor want all my ducks lined up in a row. Challenges, to me, call for imaginative solutions that come freely when I let them come by the same route and with the same assurance that I learned in music.

I have learned over many years of teaching how students bring to nursing their talents in such areas as mechanics, art, cooking, sports, sewing, painting, and so on that become ingrained in all their attempts at assessment and problem solving. Some rush for the logical solution while others take a bit more time as they examine the answer from the many angles of their art. Once you recognize just what your talents are, you can use them to develop a unique style. When you stop to acknowledge how your talents have shaped the person you are, and when you begin to see how the person you are affects your practice of nursing, you will begin to understand how you come to some of the conclusions you reach that others may not share right away. You will also gain confidence in your ability to contribute to the whole by your unique way of working through a difficult situation. So, some nurses are artistic. Others are mechanically inclined. Others have a knack for science and order. These views are synergistic, not competitive. When we are allowed to accept that our talents are gifts that we can share, nurses can come together and form practice that derives from the merger of each one's strength.

In the remainder of this part of the book, I will present the four ways of knowing as they have been developed by nurses. You can draw from each one a bit of insight that will result in a complete picture of knowledge for a healing nurse. A healing nurse bases a practice not just on the science of nursing, but how empirics, ethics, aesthetics, and personal knowledge blend together to form nursing care. For example, as we will see in the next chapter, prediction is the crown jewel of science. But prediction also flows from a greater understanding of the individual in the environment in ways that are non-empirical. One of my favorite novelists, Godwin said, "Prophecy is nothing more than seeing into the heart of what people are doing now."[10] [(240)] This quote lends credibility to the notion that without a personal understanding of the world, scientific prediction unaided would be rather limited and shallow because the underlying values and meaning embodied in the person's heart would be discounted or ignored.

Discussion and Exercises

1. Go around the room and ask each person to name a talent that she or he has. Ask the person and the group to speculate how that has influenced the nurses' practice.

2. List all the qualities and characteristics about each group member that would contribute to a unique way of practicing nursing. (Hint: see these unique facets of the person as strengths, not weakness, and remember that this discussion does not have to be deadly serious – some will provoke laughter).

Chapter IV

Understanding the World Through Empirics

For some of you, reading this chapter may feel like eating your greens before you have dessert. If I did not include it in the education of healing nurses, I would be lacking sadly in sensitivity for the role of nurses in complex situations of health care, in the same way that recommending that you eat only dessert would lead you to a lack of balance in nutrition. Taking time to explore the strengths and the limitations of empirical knowledge will put you in an excellent position to use scientific knowledge to teach others on your team about the purpose and meaning of nursing and medical research, and to understand the language that allows you to communicate with other health professionals.

Empirical knowing, the science of nursing, allows us to test a theory through research so that we can better predict the outcome of our care. The theory must come before the research, or scientists would not know how to select the factors that will be tested. For example, if we want to find a way to prevent infection, we must first understand what scientific theories tell us about what an infection is and the possible ways of transmission. As studies point to specific directions for altering care, clinical agencies can develop guidelines for care that become an official part of how care is organized and delivered in specific institutions.

According to Chinn and Kramer, the processes used in empirics are describing, explaining, and predicting. Researchers describe phenomena in detail and form explanations for the relationships between the concepts so that we can understand the phenomenon clearly. From these theories come prediction that scientists consider to be the highest form of empirical knowing. Prediction starts with a set of interrelated propositions. Let us give an example of a proposition. As a school nurse, I want to do something about violence among the school children in my district. I note that people who live in poor neighborhoods are prone to a lot more violence than people in rich neighborhoods. So I propose:

Poverty leads to violence.

This proposition spells out what I think is the relationship between poverty and violence - that it is poverty that leads to violence, not the other way around. But we obviously need a great deal more information for us to be able to accept this statement as true. And it would be a very hard proposition indeed to test because the reasons for the causality are so vague. So suppose we try to tease out a theory through developing a set of propositions that are interrelated.

1. Poverty leads to deprivation;
2. Deprivation leads to frustration;
3. Frustration leads to anger;
4. Anger leads to violence;
Therefore: **Poverty leads to violence.**

In order to test our theory of violence we could begin by testing one or more of the propositions. The proposition, frustration leads to anger, has been tested a myriad of times and reported in the social psychological literature, so we can probably assume its validity. The propositions, deprivation leads to frustration and anger leads to violence could be studied by many different methods. Even qualitative methods, such as careful observation could help lend support to the truth of these statements. The school nurse, possessing such a theory could begin to intervene into the relationship between poverty and violence. It might be unrealistic to think that a nurse could alleviate poverty, but a nurse could develop programs that would tackle many forms of deprivation and frustration that poverty forces on people.

Researchers are looking for patterns in the data, and the conclusions that they draw are based upon statistical reasoning that applies over a large sample, and that if implemented will point a nurse's practice toward productive directions. But theory based upon research findings cannot usually be applied directly to practice. Let me give you a very simple lesson in statistics.

For instance, we know that, in general, when patients get good preparation for discharge, they do better at home with their self-care. We are allowed to form this conclusion because a great many studies with good designs have shown a significant relationship between the variables of discharge planning and self-care. But in practice such a conclusion about discharge planning must be taken with more than a grain of salt, because it can only point practicing nurses toward one or more lines of action that may not be useful for every patient. Put more simply, it cannot direct practice without considering each individual patient's circumstances, because correlation based upon a research study does not mean that we have prediction in an individual case– far from it, and this is why: A correlation coefficient between two variables could be as high as 0.4 and we may find that it is significant at the 0.01 level. This is considered an excellent result in research. It means that we are very sure that when discharge planning increases, so does better self-care. But what does it really mean when applied to the outcome of self care? You can find this out if you square the correlation coefficient of 0.4:

$$0.4 \times 0.4 = 0.16$$

The result, 0.16, or the correlation coefficient squared, is called "explained variance," the percentage of self-care that explained by discharge planning. In other words, discharge planning has only explained 16 percent of self care levels. We are left with a whopping 84% of self-care that is accounted for by unknown factors.

Researchers now use sophisticated techniques that allow them to place a large number of causal variables into an equation in order to assess their effect on another variable, such as self-care. As a result, using say 10 causal factors, researchers may be able to increase prediction vastly and form better theories as they observe the order and the magnitude in the variables causing the effect. Researchers must use existing theory, some of which has not been tested in previous studies, to select the order that their variables will be entered into an equation. This step means that the research process is not actually one of objective science, but rather a complex thinking process based upon the researcher's practice and theoretical training.

Still, even using multiple causal variables, the explained variance for all factors is often not more than 50-60 percent, and many of the causes entered into the equation may be interesting, but not under the control of the nurse. For example, one factor that usually accounts for the most variance in any patient teaching situation is the patient's formal education, something that must be taken into account, but cannot be changed by nursing intervention. On the other hand, a variable such as "patient's readiness to learn," might be something a nurse could gauge and plan for by timing the intervention when the patient is ready.

Newer, better funded studies are using randomized clinical trials, meaning that patients are divided into 2 groups in which any patient has an equal chance of landing in Group E, the Experimental group or Group C, the Control group. In this design, discharge planning is performed for Group E, but not Group C. Then the results are compared. This type of study gives us better prediction because extraneous factors that might confound the results are controlled by the experimental design. Also, the experimental variable, Discharge Planning, must be spelled out in the research in such a clear way that everyone can follow it. But invariably we find as we did in the correlational design above that the findings may be more than conclusive enough to justify instituting discharge planning in your institution, but that practicing nurses must still look for many other ways, yet to be discovered, to increase after discharge self care ability, and these ways of teaching cannot be applied in a rote manner. They must be woven carefully into a complex clinical practice.

So, scientific studies can bring us closer to a knowledgeable practice that will improve care, but scientific knowledge will not replace the types of knowledge that encompass the art of nursing. It augments it by directing attention to known ways of intervening. And, it should be clear by now that scientific knowledge and practical knowledge do not exist as separate entities. Together they strengthen one another as they become entwined into a healing practice.

Whereas nurses used to be urged to utilize nursing research in practice, a newer term that has replaced the old idea of "research utilization," is *Evidence-Based Practice* (EBP). If you have not heard about EBP you will shortly. As evidence builds up in a given area about ways to approach specific patient problems, such as symptoms of delirium or dementia, research based guidelines for care can supplement, or in some cases replace the traditional ways of delivering care that were based upon opinions. But Evidence Based

Practice, unlike the old concept of research utilization, takes into account a great many factors other than research, such as patient preference and values and some of the non-empirical ways of knowing that we will discuss in the remainder of this section. [11]

Discussion and Exercises

1. What theories would be helpful as explanations for the relationship between exercise and weight gain?

2. We know that there is a positive relationship between quality of nursing care and patient recovery from surgery. List all the concepts that would account for this relationship, and attempt to interrelate these concepts as I did in the poverty-violence example above.

3. Ask someone to tell the group about a clinical situation that has them puzzled or stymied in terms of either understanding it or problem solving. Describe the phenomena in detail.

   a. What are the health consequences of the problem, including pain and suffering for the patient?

   b. Come up with one or more scientific explanations for the problem that fit with the group's diagnosis or assessment.

   c. Identify any research that would suggest ways to solve the problem, or if there is no research, what research would be needed to answer the question.

Chapter V

Understanding the World Through Ethics

Ethics is a way of knowing that arises from what we value and the moral obligations we have. For example if we value life over death, we have the obligation to promote life and prevent death, and in fact, often do it without thinking about it. According to Chinn and Kramer,[9] the processes of ethics are clarifying, valuing, and advocating. Once we identify an ethical dilemma, we must clarify our own values, learn to appreciate that there may be a number of diverse and valid values that apply to the problem, and then advocate for the best ethical solution possible, keeping in mind the patient's right to self-determination.

We achieve our moral obligations to our patients by clarifying ethics and ideals that spring from a number of social and personal foundations, and trying to implement care based upon what we think is right both overall and in that instance. It is true that right and wrong are very illusive terms, so decisions resting on values must always be revisited because one can never assume that choices that stem from these values are stable over time, even within a given individual. I will go into much more detail on this issue in Part II when I discuss existential advocacy.

Additionally, all professional groups, including the American Nurses' Association have position statements on such ethical dilemmas as assisted suicide and patient's right to self determination. It is the obligation of every licensed practitioner to be familiar with the official positions of the profession and to bring issues connected with these dilemmas to the attention of all concerned persons, including nursing staff, nursing and hospital administration, and the patient and family.

Chinn and Kramer suggest that the questions to ask oneself about a given action are: *is it right*, and *is it just*? White,[12] in her update of Carper's work adds two more critical criteria for nursing judgment: *is it good*, and *does it embody caring*? Caring allows us to go beyond the moral ideal, to a way of understanding that promotes living in the patient's world and being responsible to the patient in all decision making.

This short book on practice does not aim to teach ethics. Although it is a subject well worth pursuing, it is beyond the scope of this book to explain in depth the underlying belief system of many ethical principles such as justice, distributive justice, morality, relativism, teleology, deontology, beneficence, and so on. I do believe however, that practicing nurses should be familiar with the diverse ethical ways to approach a problem in order to be able to contribute knowledgeably as the patient's advocate during ethical grand rounds. Ethicists are usually available to the nursing staff in most inpatient institutions to provide classes and enter into nursing discussions of patient care.

But despite the lofty names of some of the ethical theories, the basic criteria for decision making are often quite practical. In employing the principles of beneficence, I am concerned with doing good, removing harm, and not inflicting harm. Among themselves, ethicists themselves employ differing criteria to problem solving, arguing whether good is effected by puzzling out the morality of every single situation individually (relativism); or if an action is good because it results in good (teleology); or whether an action can be good if it is not lawful (deontology). All are questions that we need to ask ourselves continuously as we practice. Have you ever done something for a patient that others would not approve of because the patient requested it and you were convinced that it would help the patient? How many times have you wavered between actions that you know are good and right for a patient, but that might not be allowed in your institution? Or have you ever wanted to withhold a treatment that was seemingly effective, but that you knew would not produce the outcome that the patient desired?

Ethical ways of knowing, then, are complex while appearing relatively simple. One criterion that I use all the time that I do not see mentioned in the ethics literature, is asking myself, as Plato did, when I am tempted to fudge a little bit in my duty to others: "What would happen if everyone did it?" If you can answer, "It would be fine." Then your approach may at least be harmless.

There has been hundred fold increases in medical technology and presumed medical cures. Callahan,[13] a leading medical ethicist, in discussing cultural bioethics, points out that there is no public agreement on use of technology, because there has been no public forum on how it will be used to improve individual lives and our public existence. He writes, "Far less noticed was the potent way in which biomedical innovation and medical routinization was shaping the background culture in which individual decision-making would be made."[13 (85)] In other words, the technology has been introduced that is now allowed to call the shots on morality and on ethics, but without prior discussion about how using it would affect the ethics of care. Callahan goes on to say about the consumer, "There was never, even at the start, a level playing field for the exercise of choice. The context was being manipulated by an underground culture that was both powerful and invisible."[13 (85)] Most practicing nurses are well aware of the slippery slope that medical technology presents in a large number of life and death situations, raising questions about what is life, when does it end, who should be allowed to die, and who should decide? Nurses are at the center of these debates, and the healing nurse will take on a more active role in advocating for patients.

Parker[14] shows that an ethic of care is enhanced by nurses telling stories. She states that she has never met a nurse who does not have a story to tell. Parker's own story concerned a stroke patient named "Mike," who could not move at all and could only communicate through expressions in his eyes. The worst moments in the day concerned the tremendous pain that accompanied turning, dressing change, and the wound debridements, necessitated by numerous surgeries, including amputations. Multiple systems were failing, and Mike's painful, invasive high tech treatments toward every body system were mounting in ways that only experienced nurses can know, because they have been there with hundreds of dying patients that suffer through futile medical attempts to save one organ system after another, while the patient dies like a collapsing card pack. Parker began to awaken in the middle in the night to her dreams of Mike's screams. By doing his care, and responding to the looks of pain and fear in his eyes, Parker began to understand such things as hope, courage, powerlessness, fear, suffering, and patience. Dwelling with the patient through her personal value clarification, Parker came to a tacit understanding with Mike that further medical interventions served no useful purpose for his life. She awakened to how her vision had been clouded by a training that had set her to save lives at all possible costs, including promoting suffering for Mike with ineffective treatments. Like the goddess Cassandra, who could see the truth, but would not be believed, she tried unsuccessfully to convince the physicians to really take a look at what they were doing. Her moral conflict, so familiar in nursing, was sustaining life versus self-determination. She concludes that nursing's strength is in its refusal to adopt an impartial, detached response to the ethics of care. She says, "Nurses are highly suspicious of formula ethics; they have seen too many blood sacrifices in their practice."[14 (38)]

Finally, in your efforts to determine what is ethical for your practice, no advice I could give you stands higher than that of Aristotle, who declared that virtue is not natural, but is a result of practice, like the arts. He said,

> If virtue were natural, it could not be changed by habit or teaching. It is impossible for a stone which naturally moves downhill to become habituated to moving upward; nor can any fire move downward.[15(33)]

Aristotle concluded that virtue requires doing it over and over, and as he put it, "We become harpists by playing the harp. Similarly, we become just by the practice of just actions."[15(33)]

Discussion and Exercises

1. Define to the best of your ability the term "ethics." Contrast this with "morality."

2. Discuss all the reasons why nurses are concerned with ethical principles in practice.

3. You are caring for a patient who is, by all medical assessments, terminally ill. She is experiencing pain, is bedridden, and has outlived her family and friends. She is being discharged into a nursing home to die. She begs you to help her end her life before she has to be discharged. At least, she says, don't give me anything to keep me alive

   a. What are the ethical dilemmas in either complying with or refusing her request?

   b. How would you start to examine your own values regarding what this patient is asking?

   c. How does the current health care environment either help or hinder the nurse to confront ethical dilemmas such as the one above?

Chapter VI

Understanding the World Through Aesthetics

Aesthetics is the direct experience of art - a deep, subjective experience, interpreted internally by a nurse in a way that may or may not be shared or similarly perceived by others. And like most artistic experiences, it is not expressed through language. Instead of language, aesthetics has a form, a color, a shape, or a harmony that may be beautiful or hideous.

In my work with people who were dying, I learned to appreciate the aesthetics of what I finally realized, after a time, was the art of dying. I recognized that dying, like being born, has a contour, a rhythm and a synchronization that belongs to it alone. It is not always attractive, in fact, its appearance can be downright appalling, but its configuration is always perfect for what it has to do. I can never articulate in words the art of dying, so I will not attempt it here. But because dying is an uncanny experience, I can convey to you my observations from the first time I stayed with a patient who was actively dying, through metaphor, the recounting of another uncanny experience with an art that is almost identical - when once I was stranded outdoors in an open field in the middle of one of the blinding, raging, lightening packed thunder storms that frequently come on in my home state of Texas without a second's notice, driving the temperature down 30 degrees within 5 minutes.

> The wild Texas storm – freezing cold, blinding rain, and sky-illuminating jagged electricity that extended from high in the sky all the way down to the ground, followed immediately by ear-deafening thunder - scared the hell out of me. My mind overflowed with a sense of dread, horror and excitement, and inexplicably, a grudging admiration and respect for its awesome power and destructive strength. Its terrible beauty was beyond words – a free Fourth of July spectacle like no other I had seen; only now, I was part of the firework's display. I was desperate to find shelter under a tree or in a trench, but was afraid it would lure the lightening into my path. So I had to acknowledge that what

beckoned was also dangerous. There was no place that I could run to escape, so chilled to the bone and scared witless, I plodded along, head down, in what I was hoping was in the direction of home, and prayed I would be alright. Arriving home, I breathed a sigh of relief that it was done. I was okay. I was still me.

Perhaps I could paint dying, but I am not a painter. It is enough for me that I can appreciate it first hand, not through observation, but like out in the storm, within the appalling life and death drama that is its artistic structure in real life. I cannot write the book that would allow you to borrow my aesthetic experience, but whether we participate in their creation or simply live through their effect on us, artistic interpretations of nursing phenomenon profoundly affect the way we practice nursing.

Descriptions of aesthetics in art and poetry allow us to understand processes and events that we would never otherwise be able to appreciate because we have not had a personal experience. For example, Schecter describes the aesthetic experience of pain by saying that pain is unspeakable. "It is different from death in that sense, for death, as an experience, has a voice, makes demands... if we are lucky, we may speak of our death, and if not others will speak for us."[16(123)] But in pain, we retreat into silence beyond a barrier that others cannot cross. One can only observe the grimace or the outcry. So pain has its own aesthetic experience which we can choose to grasp artistically whether we have ever been in severe pain or not.

Similarly, I arrive at a greater understanding of being incarcerated against one's will in a mental hospital through Anne Sexton's poem, *The Music Swims Back to Me*. She starts her poem with a simple question that evokes a strong response in me of bewildered, ensnared helplessness:

> *Wait, Mister. Which way is home?*
> *They turned the lights out.*[17(12)]

If Aesthetic understanding is so inexplicable that it cannot be communicated in words, then what is the purpose of discussing it as a way of knowing? Chinn and Kramer[9] convey to us that becoming nurse artists allows a process of engaging with others without placing value judgments on them, and allows us to grasp what is beyond our personal prejudices and our intellectual ways of understanding. We create our artistic practice as we try to envision bringing together everything possible to comprehend a world in a way that allows expansion of the narrow interpretations we have become conditioned to.

Consciousness expands as we move into a scene while at the same time, or even alternately, observing it from a distance. We flesh out the vision further as we participate in artistic criticism within nursing, both alone and with others in a way that gets to an implicit, consensual, and embedded understanding of human meaning that is cumulative when we bat it around together. The more we engage with different nursing subjects, the more we understand the art that is within nursing. A most vital thing that we learn to appreciate through these experiences, in the deep way we need to understand it if we are going to meet patients on their own terms, is that there is no one truth, nor does anyone own truth. Truth is much richer and more multifaceted than a single interpretation would allow, and truth takes on a personal significance when we devote time and effort to its exploration – when we accept that there are multiple, complex truths implanted in each aesthetic experience, and that they can be accessed in the same way that any art permits.

In a talk I did in Japan, boldly carrying coals to Newcastle, I borrowed a term from the major religion of the country, Buddhism, and called aesthetic phenomenon the "Zen of nursing practice." As in Zen, nurses are called upon to become ever more aware of what we are only dimly aware, by focusing on the experience of the event instead of the description. When I judge an action *empirically*, I have to separate myself from it before I can see it *objectively*. When I see it objectively, I am actually in bondage to my own theories about its nature. Experiencing through aesthetics, in tapping into an artistic mode of being, I allow myself to overcome my theoretical bias in order to blend my experience with the patient's experience to arrive at an honorable and honest conclusion. When I give myself over to the care of a patient, and experience the moment as Zen, I absorb myself completely in the task of care, moment after moment, developing a sense of the patient, and a joy of doing what needs to be done, with no thought of what I want, and no worry of meeting my own needs for power, security, and esteem. I believe that no one can expect anymore of a nurse than this.

Discussion and Exercises

1. Talk about a time when you had an aesthetic response (positive or negative) that you recognized when caring for a patient, especially one that you may not have recognized at the time. How was this experience transformative for you?

2. Discuss the various ways that practicing artistically would be a part of your ongoing learning about nursing practice. How would it change? How would you be different?

Chapter VII

Understanding the World Through Personal Knowledge

In personal knowing we use our inner experiences to understand whatever is happening in our environment. Having worked with many patients with a life threatening diagnosis, and having had a life threatening diagnosis myself, I have personal knowledge that helps me greatly in caring for persons who have been told that they have an illness that in short order could end their lives. Even though I know what the research says about stages of loss, it is personal knowing that helps me to understand the needs of someone exhibiting profound feelings of shock, fear and grief followed by depression or anger. I have a personal knowledge about the broader meaning of what it means to experience loss of health and potential loss of life. Shakespeare observed that if we know ourselves, and are true to ourselves, we cannot be false to others. In nursing, this means that authentic understanding of those under our care starts with a deep commitment to our own self-knowledge and truth.

So personal knowing is realized through experience, but we must attune our ears and our hearts to learn from experience. The fact that we might have experienced something similar to the patient does not mean that we have allowed ourselves to understand it in a way that it can be drawn on in care. Utilizing personal knowledge then requires a process of self understanding or self truth that leads one to consider one's own experiences and experience of others in the deepest possible way.

Consequently, according to Chinn and Kramer,[9] the first step in the processes of personal knowing is centering - opening oneself up through centering clears our minds of the prejudice that prohibits a focus on the meaning of the experience. Then finally we engage in a process of realizing. In realizing, we consider the broader meaning of the experience as it applies to many life situations. So in personal knowing, we are true to ourselves when we listen carefully enough to hear out entirely our own experience and that of others. This process promotes self-knowledge that is free of so many protective emotions that we usually employ to guard ourselves from painful growth, a growth that cannot occur unless we allow in multiple interpretations that replace the constricted views that we usually content ourselves with. When centering ourselves, we permit into our often closed minds the voice of the experience at hand and allow that voice to be heard in a way that will overcome the rigid thinking that usually has its hold on us. Finally, personal knowing involves expanding into an authentic, genuine self as we make that experience part of who we are.

To illustrate the process of personal knowing described above, I gave students in my classes an exercise that was rather frustrating for them, but one that they never forgot. I developed a short case study that was based on a true event. In it, I describe a sick and dying 90 year old man who has had advanced vascular disease resulting in above the knee amputations of both his legs. With his 87 year old wife's help and a little help from a home health agency, he has been living at home. He has become more despondent and confused. He gets angry at his wife when tasks are not done perfectly, or things are not set on the table beside his bed in the exact order he likes them. He is frightened when alone, even when his wife goes out for a few minutes to shop for food, and begs not to be left. When we meet the patient, he has been admitted to the hospital with a lower G.I. blockage that has resulted in a colostomy. Mentally, he is very confused and disoriented.

His wife appears quite frail and exhausted. She tells the nurse that she is worn out from 24 hour care of her husband resulting in lack of adequate sleep and rest. She never gets more than 30 minutes of sleep without interruption. She refuses the hospital nurse's efforts to teach her to care for the colostomy, because she says that she cannot even manage what she has to do now. The couple has limited sources of family support, because their adult children, who live very far away, can participate in planning, and they can make frequent visits to help in crisis, but they cannot be there all the time. The couple many times has refused offers to move nearer their children, preferring to stay in the community they have always lived in. Neither will hear of going to a retirement center that has a range of medical services. They will stay in their home until they die. All their friends are becoming old and sick as they are, and are of limited help. A major dilemma is that the wife wants the husband to be discharged to a geriatric center until he is stable, but he begs to go home, and won't hear of any other plan for discharge.

I put the students in small groups to discuss how they would respond to this couple. Having used this case study for a few years, I was always interested in the facts that everyone added to what was written, and also that students simply ignored many of the facts as they discussed what knowledge one would need to help the couple through this period. Obviously, I have biased the facts the most because I have chosen what to include in the case study. In doing so, I was wholly guided by my past experience and the values that struck me when analyzing this case.

Similarly, the past experiences of the students pointed their observations and interpretations in definite directions. Women who had experienced care of a sick husband, or whose mothers had taken care of their fathers, had a very different take on what was "really going on between this couple" than those who had no personal knowledge of the problems that families have in home care for the sick and elderly. Some were quick to blame the wife or the husband for not planning ahead, or not anticipating the problems of this stage of life. Still others tried to manufacture family, friends, or other resources where they did not exist. "There must be someone to help," they would declare, hopefully. Others had negative views of geriatric centers and what they are for, and insisted that the wife should be able to handle the problem, rather then having to resort to such a drastic solution. Others had strong views about the exploitation of women in the family, surmising that the husband had always dominated the wife and demanded her total attention to his welfare at the risk of her own health and welfare. They would stop their conversations to come and ask me if I had more information in a certain area, but I would not give it to them, reminding them that they already had more information than nurses usually do when making care assessments.

So lacking complete information, students would try to fill in the gaps in knowledge with their personal experience, and even when they had the facts, they weighed the significance of these facts through the screen of their own experience. Rarely did anyone recognize how much their personal knowledge affected their interpretations of clinical data. In analyzing the case in class, some students threw empirical knowledge to the wind. They wanted the husband to go home, even without good colostomy care, if it must be. Home is the place to be, they argued, and who is to say that they are wrong? In looking at the same data, some students were drawn to the ethical issues that separate the will and the rights of the husband from those of the wife. Joining either side seemed wrong to them, and they sought for a way to satisfy everyone's needs, or at least to take everyone's values into account. Opinions abounded, but in this case study, which is very typical of the plight of many elderly people, many students began to feel angry and frustrated when solutions could not be found. They were angry at the lack of social and medical choices that put people into this dilemma in the first place. Some were furious with a medical model that cuts away people's body parts, little by little, with the predictable results that they now see before them.

Then, after hearing all the opinions that the small groups reported, I asked them to go back into their groups; to stop arguing for their own point of view in order to listen and learn from each other's personal knowing and sense of what is right and good. Also, I asked them to hear, as well as they could, what the facts in the case study might be requiring of them personally. I could tell they thought they had already talked this case to death and were reluctant to spend more time on it. But in sustained "talking and listening sessions" concerning the case of the elderly man and woman, what at last came to light, was a sense of a profound and intense phenomenological understanding of the experience, not only the experience of the couple under discussion, but of the complexity of the issues that nursing is charged to deal with daily, and how our superficial thinking can distort and mislead us into believing that easy answers will become acceptable solutions for other people's complex lives.

Students learned to project themselves into the suffering of the husband and wife and their adult children. Instead of anger at the elderly couple and the family for not solving their problems, they saw how health care rules have worked against rational problem-solving. They learned that what they hold dear may not be the right solution for everyone; what they have experienced may not be the experience of others. Yet they also saw that lived experience is their only tool if they hope to understand fundamental life dilemmas enough to be helpful to patients. They became clearer from discussing this situation about the need for a nursing approach that values advocacy and caring for people in the shape and form that they present themselves to us for help.

This clinical example is not unique in nurse's practice. All our patients need us to be able to draw on a diverse, collective knowledge base that can aid in solving intricate problems in ways that are clinically sound and non-judgmental. All patients need nurses who can consider fully their complicated lives, and develop approaches that are aimed at overcoming the personal, organizational, and social constraints that have increasingly caused us to put the bottom line ahead of patient needs.

When these students entered the course, many were sure that the practice of nursing must be weighted firmly in the direction of better research and improving practical nursing tasks. When they emerged from the course, I observed a broadening of this one-sided approach toward an understanding that practice involves much more than science or tasks, extending to who the nurse is, who the patient is, and how emerging personal knowledge sets down the rules for the seemingly simple act of caring for a patient and a patient's family.

The Art of Becoming a Nurse Healer

Discussion and Exercises

1. Use the above case study, or one that you are dealing with now to express your personal understanding about the dilemma of the patient and the family.

2. Discuss one personal experience that you have had that might impact positively or negatively on how you interpret the data in this case study.

3. How does opening up to experience authenticate a nursing approach to a complex patient situation?

4. Chinn and Kramer recommend journaling as a way to improve personal knowing. How can your group incorporate journaling to improve patient care?

Part 2

The Nature of a Caring Relationship

Something we were withholding made us weak,
Until we discovered it was ourselves.
We were withholding from our land of living. [18]
--Robert Frost

The philosopher, Noddings[19] writes that caring is not some tender-minded activity. Like a bear with a cub, nurses are hard-wired to protect furiously what we are responsible for. A great deal of mental and emotional toughness is required for caring, protection, and advocacy. No cowards need apply. But more basically, can any nurse possibly think that caring is actually a choice when we realize that the alternative to caring is not caring? In this section, I will talk about the essential aspects of a helping relationship, including some of the barriers. Happily the empowerment that comes out of caring is mutual, so when a nurse is in a caring relationship with a patient, both are renewed. As Frost said in the above quote, withholding makes us weak. The outcome of investing yourself in another, whether it is a personal or professional relationship, is a surge in your own growth and energy.

In this section, you will learn how to avoid role entrapment, a major barrier to a healing relationship. You will have an opportunity to discover how to put yourself in the best state of mind to care for others within a nurse-patient relationship. Finally, you will learn the importance of a role that is exceedingly complicated– advocacy. Although much has been written about advocacy and empowerment, there has been a general lack of acknowledgment about how incredibly difficult it is for nurses to enact it.

Chapter VIII

Role Entrapment: Barrier to a Healing Relationship

Nurses are among the most popular and respected of all professionals. Almost everyone would agree that having access to nursing care is an enormous comfort to anyone in sickness and distress. That is the heart of what we do. But I believe that the sort of helping relationship that so many professionals form with patients is not helpful at all. The model of helping that most of us learned is fraught with traps for the helper, who may go away thinking, "What I did was so useful to this patient," while the patient feels devalued by professional self-importance and by the hierarchy of power that seems to go with helping. Dass and Gorman warn,

> The most familiar models of who we are – father and daughter, doctor and patient, helper and helped – often turn out to be major obstacles to the expression of our caring instincts; they limit the full measure of what we have to offer one another.[20 (28)]

From my own experience, I have concluded that this statement is true. When we offer professional advice it often falls on deaf ears because we have assumed that patients will conform to the rather restricted patient role that we have placed them in and it will be enough for them to stay there while we play out our limited professional parts. Thus "role entrapment" is a major barrier to helping another that must be confronted by every nurse who wants to care.

When we meet a physician or a nurse at a party, they are just ordinary folk who act like everyone else and talk about the same things everyone talks about. In other words, they are whole people at the party – individuals who do not limit themselves to the professional persona that they put on in patient care. Putting on their professional garb, they morph into something else entirely, hiding behind a busy facade of authority that provides an impenetrable barrier on a human level.

Within a relationship when one person plays out a professional role, it limits greatly the role of the other person. So, the more you think of yourself in the role of a nurse, the more pressure there is on someone else to be a patient. The more a person becomes a patient, the more passive and compliant they become. In acute settings, in which all that is required are emergency measures for life saving or brief instructions on short-term treatment, role entrapment is not so evident, although it is present. But in chronic illness which comprises most of the health care burden in this country, patients may be limited to patient-hood for the rest of their lives – the amputee diabetic in your primary care practice; the blind woman in room 305. And these patients may be in contact, over a life time, with helpers who carry out a professional role with very little cognizance of how being regarded as a patient can wear away another person's ability to be a human being, rather than "blind" or "disabled." Consequently, patient confidence may be eroded systematically over a number of encounters, as professionals begin to assume authority over their very lives, a state which is disempowering, dehumanizing, and controlling, and over many years may have a devastating effect on identity.

In my specialty of nursing, mental health, I have found that psychiatric patients rarely, if ever, come into a relationship with a nurse expecting to be empowered, because in that field especially we regard the patient, not as a person, but as a mental illness.[21] Patients with chronic mental illness who are experiencing a return of symptoms, put off presenting themselves for care for as long as they can because they dread returning to a role in which they are devalued, stripped of their humanness, and told what to do and when to do it from morning until night.

But role entrapment is hardly limited to psychiatry. In my studies and clinical practice with persons with HIV disease, I found similar attitudes among helping professionals. These patients too, were treated as a disease and their lives were commandeered in order to introduce treatments that patients sometimes did not welcome or desire, although they might have if someone had taken the time to explore the patient's values before demanding compliance to a treatment.

I learned after awhile that most of my patients had become apt students of their disease. They could reel off facts and figures from research studies that involved effectiveness and side effects of various treatments as well or better than I could. What they often wanted from me was an active, knowledgeable sounding board to try out their ideas on, and someone to raise the critical questions important for decision making. They made decisions based upon the state of the science combined with their own beliefs, their goals, and their aspirations for their lives. Many were working in satisfying jobs or going to school to earn degrees for which they were proud, while many of their families and caregivers wanted them to limit their lives by staying home and taking it easy.

Patients often had established personal health regimes that they had confidence in, but about which we professionals had no interest at all. These health efforts may or may not have met the criteria for scientific veracity, but they were highly important for the patient. One man, for example, had been on a very strict, nearly unworkable diet to control bowel and other symptoms. He told me one day that he was now eating most everything he wanted because he had discovered that when he blessed his food, it did not harm him. What would have been the result had I corrected him with the information that there is no scientific proof of the usefulness of his blessing to prevent diarrhea?

In this same clinic, 20 men in late stages of HIV decided to go off their medications in order to travel to Brazil to take part in a treatment designed by a Korean doctor, who believed he could help them with sparse whole grain and vegetable diet and a set of very difficult exercises. This invitation did not seem to be a scam as he was not only paying their airfare to Brazil, where they would go for treatment, but also was not charging them for the treatment, food, or lodging. I was in much trepidation about them doing this, and told them so. Yet, it would be impossible not to see the hope and the enthusiasm that this venture generated at a time when the only anti HIV drug available was AZT, a drug that had exceedingly serious and life-limiting side effects, but was not especially effective in holding off the rampage of the virus for very long. These men knew well the facts of their disease and what they were risking. But this was balanced with their understanding of their dim prognosis with treatment, given current medical knowledge. They felt accurately that they had no future life, and that they deserved this chance at health. At their invitation, I attended some of the exercise periods they held to ready themselves for the trip to Brazil. These yoga-like poses were so difficult that I, a healthy, fit person, struggled with them. Nevertheless these very sick, but plucky individuals persisted, to my great admiration. Their attitude was, "I want go out of this life fighting," and who could blame them. Should I have put on my professional cloak, crossed my arms in front of my chest, and lectured to them about the danger of going off their drugs, when they knew the consequences better than I?

Nevertheless the medical board in that state, assuming resident authority over the lives of these patients, began to take steps to bar them by a court injunction from traveling out of the country. There turned out to be so many legal delays, that attempts to restrict "their patients" were unsuccessful. It was fortunate that the attempt at a legal ban was ineffective, because when the men returned, incredibly all were in better health as indicated by weight gain, greatly increased t-cell counts, and enormous increases in energy and self-confidence. Even though I could not have predicted this outcome, I supported them and helped to ease their journey as much as I could. I believe that just because someone wears the label of patient does not mean that they cannot embrace other ways of healing that I may not understand or condone. In my caring of them, I came to recognize that they very much had the right to find ways to be the best they could be.

Role entrapment impedes helping because instead of viewing a patient as a whole person who often has a great deal of knowledge, and who is entitled to a set of rights and responsibilities, such as the right to self determination and the right to lead a rich life despite the illness, we persist in seeing the person as a disease, a symptom, or a treatment. We foster the sick role, by protecting the treatment instead of supporting the full lives they are here on earth to live. This narrow attitude is especially devastating over time, and the greater the debilitation, the greater is the robbing of identity and self-worth. Many long term survivors of chronic illness establish their own care routines based on reading and information gleaned from support groups - practices that they believe keep them healthy and functioning. I know from experience that when such patients come in for care they keep silent about many of the forms of treatment outside mainstream medicine that they have accessed in order to avoid the standard lectures on inappropriate treatments that they do not welcome.

I believe, too that most patients tend to keep most personal information to themselves. There is no need to present oneself as an intact human being with hopes and dreams if nobody cares. Most times it goes better for patients if we know nothing about them personally at all –if they never expect to be treated as a whole person by helpers who regard themselves as whole persons. We are all in tight roles, and patients will be less frustrated if they just surrender to their patient-hood and get it over with. They submit to becoming their medical history and their current illness with their symptoms, allergies to drugs, and the many other questions on the intake exam. But as Dass and Gorman[20] put it, we cannot really believe that we are "nobody" either. That just does not work, and the primary reason that it does not is that there are so many decisions to be made about treatment and care that just cannot be decided on the medical facts alone. Any "herd mentality" that works against individuality also snuffs out empowerment and the resulting good decision making.

Another pitfall of role entrapment is how easy it is to use our knowledge to label and judge without taking into account the patient's point of view on what the problem is. Mitchell[22] describes an elderly patient, Mrs. T who was given the psychological label of "hoarder" because she kept the plastic medicine cups that the nurses brought her pills in. She stacked them on the table beside her bed, and did not allow the nurses to remove them. The nursing staff labeled this as "hoarding behavior," and discussed how to break her of it. Mitchell, a clinical specialist, went to see the patient after the nurses had already come in and thrown out all her hoarded cups. The patient was understandably upset, since she felt that this behavior was not hurting anyone. Mrs. T said, "I was just keeping them because as the days passed, I watched the stack get higher and higher. When I looked at the cups, I knew something about myself – the days I spent here." [(175)] After hearing her out, Mitchell realized that this behavior, so abhorrent and strange to the nurses, was simply Mrs. T's very creative way of structuring her time. After that the nurses let her keep her cups. This incident reminded me another patient, Jim, who structured his time that way. Each morning the newspaper was delivered with a rubber band around the paper. Jim saved the rubber bands and made them into a ball to mark the time when he would be through with his chemotherapy treatment. He joked that when it was large enough to bounce, he would be finished. Luckily Jim did not have to contend with the nurses that were described in Dr. Mitchell's article to throw out his rubber ball, because he told me he thoroughly enjoyed throwing it against the wall when he was finished with treatment. Each rubber band was a day that he gave to his recovery.

The best advice I can offer on avoiding role entrapment is to examine your own intentions during care, asking yourself if you are objectifying patients as you care for them. In the introduction to this book, I talked about approaching strangers as though they were your own family. We treat family members and friends as though they are real people who are part of us. So trying to determine for each patient the answer to the question, "Who are you?" will set you in a mind frame to go beyond patient-as-object, to a human-to-human healing relationship.

Discussion and Exercises

1. Describe a time when you were torn between your role as a nurse and your human feelings about care of a patient?

2. Use the example in the text about the HIV patients who went to Brazil to identify the professional conflicts that you would have had in this situation. How would you have tried to solve these conflicts?

3. Discuss a time when a label or a description of a patient or a patient's behavior that was mentioned in report or by another nurse influenced negatively your care of a patient. How could you handle that constructively?

The Caring Relationship

Patients are vigilant in their observations of their caregivers, always watching and listening for the word or sign that will enhance hope and recovery or the opposite - herald impending morbidity or debilitating disease. The patient interprets every detail of the nurse-patient interaction as either helpful or not helpful, no matter when it happens in the course of an illness. Patients also judge us in terms of our caring by the way that we establish our presence with them, even before we say one word. The results of the patient's evaluation of our intentions are often quite visible in the patient's response to illness and healing.

I know from my own clinical experience and that of countless of my students that patients pay close attention to the clues we put out. They become experts at interpreting the behavior of their care-givers. The minute you walk into their presence they ask themselves, "Can I trust this one?" The fact that this information is also used by them to assess their own ability to recover at your hands makes it vital that a healing nurse convey interest, presence, and hope. Although there is still scientific debate about whether there is a direct, positive relationship between the patient's belief and the patient's recovery, we must act as if whatever information that patients obtain about themselves under our care may affect the patient's health, assisting to move the patient along the road to either ill health or good health. And I think we can all agree that a fearful and frightened patient will not be in the best position to heal.

The hospital and the clinic that are so familiar and safe for us, are very frightening places for outsiders. To patients they are a maze of impersonal and busy personnel, scary machines, and incomprehen-sible procedures. The horror exists that amidst all these unfamiliar and alien practices, they will get lost in the shuffle, or that something vital will be missed, and too often their fears are realized. This point was brought home dramatically to me by one of my PhD students, a critical care clinical specialist. She decided to follow up with some of the patients after they went back to the general floors to see if they could say what it was about the nursing care that was important to them. One man, Bill, told this story:

> When I left CCU to return to the regular floor, I was terrified. I was sure I would die now because nobody would be monitoring me as closely. I would just be left to die. I had begged to remain in the CCU for at least a day longer. I remembered from before, the busy nurses who barely had time to put their heads in the door. Just after they transferred me to my bed, a nurse stuck her head in and said, "Well it's about time you got here. I have been waiting for you. Let's see if we can get you comfortable and start you on the road back to going home." When she said that, I just felt wonderful. She stayed and took my blood-pressure and temperature, and made sure I was comfortable. She showed me my call light, and then left, telling me to let her know if I needed anything. I felt peaceful for the first time since I knew I was being discharged from CCU. I knew then that I was going to be okay.[23]

Similarly, Montgomery tells a story about a cardiac patient for whom the nurse performed a caring act that was so simple, but in doing it, she turned the patient's life around. Despairing of his ability to withstand his surgical treatment, the patient said, "I'm no hero, I just can't go through with this." The nurse responded vehemently: "Heroes are ordinary people faced with extraordinary circumstances, and instead of running away, they stand and face whatever the circumstance is!" Montgomery reported, "The patient repeated this statement many times, and credited her with getting him through the experience. He did well with his surgery and recovery and was out of the hospital quickly."[24] [(23)] The nurse in this story cared enough not to accept the patient's pessimism and defeat. Her simple intervention was both impassioned and intensely caring on behalf of a patient's life. Patients are often looking for excuses to drop their negative mind-set toward their own healing. Their negativity is created out of fear, not desire. Even very tiny interventions can disrupt this destructive pattern.

If caregivers do not intervene in crucial conversations in order to deliver challenges to a patient's doubts; if they do not lend support to the often latent strengths needed to overcome defeatist attitudes, recovery is retarded sometimes until it is almost too late. I am not talking about sugary phrases such as, "Everything will be fine." The healing nurse listens for the small spark that heralds a beginning positive attitude and lends her or his strength to support the healthy part of the patient. The healing nurse searches for ways to convey to the patient an attitude of "I am in this battle with you."

"But I don't have time to practice like that," I hear you saying. Of course you do not have a lot of unencumbered time, but I remind you that a nurse that does not have time to care does not have time to be a nurse. In contrast to the lack of time argument, I find the most compelling and valid case for caring in the realization that there is no objective justification for the idea that caring takes more time than not caring.[25] Caring is not an action, *per se*, but a state of mind and an attitude. Above, in the case of Bill who was terrified to transfer out of CCU, the nurse took less than one minute to size up the situation and convey a caring interest by her welcoming manner, a few short sentences, and her body and facial language, indicating she was engaged.

But, in a busy inpatient situation, even if it took a few minutes longer would you rather answer the patient's call button four times, or take care of the concern while you are there? In a busy clinic where you are limited to 15 minutes per patient, would you rather take care of the issue or have the patient return to your primary care practice every week? As an example of the latter, a medical resident in a university practice requested that Janice Lawson, an FNP student in one of my classes, take over the care of a woman who was given the most unwarranted label of, "high crock index." He was tired of this patient coming to the outpatient clinic every week with vague and formless complaints, and wanted her off his list. Although the nurse had a busy caseload too, she decided that on the first visit she could justify spending more time than the 15 minutes allowed to find out what was going on to see if she could get to the bottom of the physical complaints. After a half hour of intensive listening and a physical examination, Ms. Lawson made a diagnosis of mild to moderate depression. The patient lived far from her family and was married to a merchant marine who was gone for 6 months at a time. She had nobody to turn to. She did not know what she needed, or how to inform the busy resident as to what was happening to her.

Her vague complaints were her efforts to obtain help in a care system that was only geared to investigating immediate medical problems. The patient experienced relief just from talking and the nurse's caring interventions. Then Ms. Lawson arranged further help from psychiatry and social services. When she followed up with a phone call in a month, the patient's depression was lifting and the physical problems had cleared up entirely. The patient continued her anti-depressants, but otherwise no longer needed to rely on the medical clinic for care.

Skilled caring practitioners learn to establish a caring and listening presence with patients in the space of a few minutes. In one study, conducted at the University of Texas at Austin, we found that patients judged a nurse's caring intent in the first second of interaction.[26] They seemed to have an immediate sixth sense about who would care, and who would be there if they were needed. This assessment even extended to whom they could trust if they had an emergency or when they were being administered drugs, if they were getting the correct drug and dosage. Indeed, they rated nurses they assessed as having a caring attitude higher on their ability to do technical tasks. Having made a positive assessment about a nurse's caring of them, they were able to be relaxed when a nurse was doing her or his job, and also when the nurse was not there in actual physical presence, they felt comforted and cared for. Patients believed that this relaxed state contributed to their eventual recovery.

It should be apparent from all the above examples that empathy is crucial for caring. Without empathy, we could never put ourselves in a position to allow another's experience to guide our actions. But empathy goes far beyond just trying to appreciate what a patient feels by imagining what it would be like for you. That would be an intellectual exercise, much too easy a route for a healing nurse, because it would not touch you or your life at all. In fact, empathy really means projecting yourself into the world of the other person in order to understand what an experience means to someone else. Such a projection creates a fundamental respectful stance that allows an authentic connection with others, even others that we are not particularly fond of.

The poet, Ann Sexton,[27] in lecturing to her class on the lyric instances that flow from poetry, challenged the class to view a rapist empathetically. For most of us, a rapist is not someone we want to get to know in any shape or form, so her challenge presents a most difficult exercise in empathy. A rapist perpetrates abhorrently violent acts on others that they never forget; he creates a horrific harm that most victims never completely recover from; he gratifies his own needs for power and control with thoughtless regard for the women's or men's lives he is harming. Once you find out that a person is a rapist, this is such an overwhelming identity that the rest of the person's character does not matter. So how do you form an empathic relationship with such a person, such a human being who might come under your care as a nurse? Would you refuse to care for him? Would you give the care, but withhold all but the most essential of services?

Confronting this sort of dilemma empathetically, by projection of yourself, means trying to see a patient who has done an act that you cannot accept in as many diverse ways as you can. Sexton suggests that you write his biography. In this biography, you look for him in a coffee shop having a cup of coffee and a clam roll. Then realizing that you like coffee and clam rolls, too, you have a start on seeing that you have something in common with a rapist. Sexton writes, "I myself like clam rolls, but I have more than a clam roll in common with the rapist. What have I ever wanted to take? When have I ever wanted to terrify?"[27(358)] Hence, empathy suspends judgment temporarily by erasing separation. I do not mean for you to take out of this chapter that you need to find a rapist to love, or count rapists among your friends, or take a rapist home and embrace him into your life. This is not only unnecessary, it would not be good for you. Rapist here is used as a symbol for the way that we use identity to label, and how we pick out the worst thing that a person has ever done to judge the whole person. I can confess here and now that I would not want to be known for the worst thing I ever did. Would you? But uncaring nurses do this with patients all the time. I have heard it in the nurses' station, and so have you. Remember that any of us can love the lovable. It takes the effort of a nurse healer to find ways to love the unlovable, and we are called upon to do this in every nursing encounter, for we are often seeing people at their very worst.

In Western society, we learn to objectify other people in a way that indicates that they are unconnected to us. Self-in-relation, an idea that Allan and I wrote about several years ago, expounds the idea that if we choose to be whole people, we cannot exist as separate little souls, trying to maintain life while rootless from our sources of support.[3] We are all part of the same universe and energy field. For that reason, we become caring people though a process of self-empowerment that allows us to value our own life as a part of an integrated whole of universal lives. When we approach patients as empowered, spiritual nurses, who have a sense of the meaning of our own lives and our connections with others, we become free to step out of the constricted world we have built for ourselves, and only then can we allow ourselves to wander fearlessly into the unknown suffering of patients. Knowing the value and meaning of our own lives becomes the catalyst to exploring what is possible in the time and space surrounding us. So we open up to the possibility of a healing world in which each gives all that he or she has to others and expects the same reciprocity from them. Making connections becomes a cyclical process in that as empowered nurses we learn to connect with patients, and then in our connections, we find surges of growth in further self-empowerment.

Although in Part III, I will cover some techniques that will aid you in helping patients to achieve their own goals for recovery, caring in itself is not an array of techniques that can be taught. Rather it is a set of attitudes and behaviors that you bring to work every day that can be laid out as guidelines for integration of caring into your nursing tasks. It is your belief in yourself as a competent person who can make a difference, along with your courageous willingness to engage others in a caring act that results in a healing outcome. There are some specific caring beliefs and behaviors that can be identified from the literature that I will cover in Part III that will help you to convey caring, but spontaneous acts of caring that flow from the heart of the nurse to the heart of the patient are not replaceable by techniques. I said in the beginning that caring takes toughness, and a great part of that toughness involves your efforts to enter intrepidly into another's world —be it a patient, a colleague, a friend, family member, or stranger, without thought of what you are going to get out of it, and with no thought of what people will think of you. Believe me, though, you will get a great deal in return over time. Caring always rebounds back onto the one caring. But if you say a caring word to someone and get rebuffed or it elicits a hostile response, instead of allowing yourself to feel hurt or sorry that you cared, remember that a grateful reply is not what you are looking for. Instead, caring is the virtue you are seeking in yourself. So when you care, you are true to yourself, and you can never be wrong.

Discussion and Exercises

1. Describe a time when your caring or the caring of another nurse made a difference for a patient. Describe the caring behavior and the outcome.

2. Discuss a full definition of empathy. Come up with as many ways of describing empathy as you can. Give some clinical examples of this concept in action.

Chapter X

Advocacy

In almost every basic nursing text there is at least one sentence declaring that a nurse should be an advocate for the patient. And why not? Nurses are knowledgeable and we do our work in the direct presence of patients. The intimate relationship we have with patients and families puts nurses in a position to hear confidences and concerns that they would never bring up with a physician. But all my experience has taught me that advocacy is among the most difficult of nursing roles to actually carry out.

Nurses are not generally independent practitioners, but are employees of health care organizations that frequently use paternalistic decision making patterns that hold little value for patient empowerment. Nurses are not only captive to these restricted moral standards, but after a time our own values are eroded and we come to accept them. Which treatment decisions get implemented depends on the power structure in the care team as well as many personal characteristics of the patient, including age, social status, amount of support from family, and degree of assertiveness.

Advocacy as a term is poorly understood. Gadow,[28] a nurse philosopher, and a major contributor to our thinking in this area, has written definitive articles showing that advocacy is best understood as a way of interacting with patients or families that helps them arrive at a decision that is good for them. Calling this form of advocacy *existential advocacy*, Gadow says that patients can only make an informed decision when they have all the facts and when they have adequate support to sift through a thought process that aims to explore their beliefs and wishes. In actual practice though, providers decide what is good for a patient based upon accepted, universal criteria that steer the patient in the direction of making the "right" choice. The outcome is often a resolution that is right for the provider, but not for the patient. To give a really personal example here, when I was diagnosed with cancer 22 years ago, the rules at University of California, San Francisco stated that patients, with their families, had the right to visit the three types of physicians who had treatments to offer a cancer patient: surgical, medical, and radiation oncologists. As I made my rounds, I could not help but observe that each of these specialists was geared only to their own area of expertise, touting the impressive results they had achieved, and trying to push me in the one direction, while subtly demeaning and discounting results accomplished by the other two. Given how differently they interpreted the evidence, I began to wonder if they were all living on the same planet, much less inhabiting offices in the same medical school. Turning to my nursing colleagues was no help either, as they each had their own views of treatment that they were trying to push me toward. I ended up making my own lonely decision, and as it turned out, I have never been really happy with it. Some knowledgeable person could have stepped in to help me sort out what I needed, but nobody did. I ended up going with the providers that I liked the best.

Gadow writes that *paternalism* is a form of advocacy which, "is the use of coercion in order to provide a good that is not desired by the one whom it is intended to benefit."[28(82)] More importantly, in most of the cases of paternalistic care that nurses witness, patients are not even given the alternatives in a way that would allow collaborative decision making. Another minimal form of advocacy is *consumerism*, in which we present to the patient the entire array of choices and leave it to the patient to make the decision.[28] Consumerism does not go far enough in helping another person decide what is best and right in that individual case and what will fit into the patients stated values. Yet, even consumer advocacy is lacking when patients are not even exposed to all the alternatives with a fair and honest assessment of their benefits and harms.

The type of advocacy I experienced was a combination of consumerism and paternalism. I was exposed to the alternatives, but not in a way that would hand over to me the full evidence needed to make an informed decision, nor did anyone help me to sort out my own values. Despite the reams of words written about patient empowerment, consumerism/paternalism has been the foundation for patient decision making in health care since the first white coat was donned and the first stethoscope installed in the pocket. Medical entitlement to patient ownership is so well accepted in health care that questions are no longer raised about its existence, and if they are, little action is taken to sanction practitioners who limit patient rights by persuasion or intimidation. In my own practice with persons with terminal and life threatening illness, I have seen how reluctant patients are to disagree with providers, even when the patient feels adamant about not selecting a type of treatment. Patients will accept prescriptions and then not fill them. They will fill prescriptions and not take the drug. Sometimes they will just abscond, preferring to leave before they will disagree. A bright light on the horizon can be found in the recent literature on shared decision making which promotes a style of provider-patient interaction that is balanced and supportive to patient rights and patient empowerment.[29]

I probably do not have to convince the healing nurse that empowerment is the cure for the problem of paternalism, but it is a sad truth that nurses must be cautious in providing patients with avenues for empowerment in the face of a situation in which another provider with more power is determined to steer the patient along only one course. I have heard of more than one nurse who has been taken to task or fired for providing information on other, well accepted courses of treatment, or sanctioned when he or she listened to a patient's doubts and encouraged the person to talk it over with family and other providers. Writing about toxic organizations, Porter-O'Grady and Malloch[30] discuss a nurse who put her own job on the line to report a powerful consulting physician to the attending physician when the consult instituted a treatment that violated the stated wishes of a patient and family. They talk about how difficult this line of action was and how risky was her stance. To them though, this sort of intervention, even as admirable as it is, does not go far enough. They write:

> Advocacy leadership in health care is a proactive process. Its purpose is to create the conditions for patients to receive the care they desire. It involves much more than removing the barriers as they are identified; in fact, the goal of advocacy leadership is to avoid having barriers in the first place. [30 (241)]

Existential Advocacy, shared decision making, and advocacy leadership comprise the gold standard of advocacy when embedded into the framework of the organization, and in a way that assures that there is the highest value placed on respecting patient rights to self-determination. Such a stance involves a great commitment on the part of all concerned because it is not a simple process in which information is passed from provider to patient. Advocacy involves a process of empowerment that is aimed at helping another reach his or her full potential.[31] In taking leadership for advocacy the nurse healer is required to become part of the patient's life for a short time, to be with the patient in a subjective way.

Gadow says that we can only discover certain data from patients through reflecting on our own experiences, not through objective knowledge. She directs us to enter the patient's world through embodying their suffering as we experience it in light of our own lives. When we approach patients in this way, we cannot be unmoved by their pain because we are now on familiar terms, body to body, with how suffering feels. Recently, one of my neighbors had a severe and persistent case of flu with raging body aches, high fever, splitting headache, diarrhea, and vomiting. She conjectured that if this is how she would feel for the rest of her life, she would rather die because life would not be worth living in such acute pain and suffering. Then she said, "Lying there, I reflected upon my mother's refusal to take further chemotherapy at the end of her life. At the time, I so much wanted her to do it, but now for the first time I see why she refused. She had had enough."

In existential advocacy, patients can move through steps in decision making with another person who is clearly on their side, not advocating in a biased way or holding onto a hidden agenda of which the patient is unaware. Advocacy cannot be enacted by nurses who are lone rangers in paternalistic organizations. Nurse healers need the support of colleagues all along the hierarchy of the organizational structure. This support can only be gained when nurses are exposed to the issues involved in advocacy and then encouraged to discuss them as they apply to specific patient situations. I do not intend to convey that advocacy is an impossible role, but clearly it is a very difficult one. I will talk more about ways to overcome some of the obstacles to becoming an advocate in Chapter 13 when I discuss the environment for caring.

Discussion and Exercises

1. Describe an actual patient situation from your past or present practice.

   a. What would be the nursing intervention for the 3 types of advocacy described: Paternalism, consumerism, existential advocacy?

   b. What are the barriers in your practice setting to existential advocacy?

   c. What can be done to remove these barriers entirely or modify them?

2. List all the support you might have in enacting leadership advocacy? How can nurses work to increase this support, to insure that no nurse will take a stand without support?

3. Give your own example of a patient situation in which advocacy was needed instead of what appeared to be right medically.

Part 3

Nurse Healing in Action

*Give us back our suffering, we cry to Heaven in our hearts –
suffering rather than indifferentism; for out of nothing comes
nothing. But out of suffering may come the cure.
Better have pain than paralysis!
-Florence Nightingale[32] [(29)]*

As you learned in Part 2 of this book, a most important caring role of a healing nurse is participating in the art of deep engagement in the suffering of the patient. Over time, the withholding of caring, or what Nightingale calls indifferentism, has a very dismal side effect. As she said in the quote above, nothing comes of it, at least not anything positive. A non-caring nurse will eventually be a victim of burnout, a sad state of affairs in which a nurse, having withdrawn from caring responsibilities, becomes cynical, contemptuous, discontented, and angry before finally dropping out. Nurses do not burn out because they have cared too much, but because they have invested too little.[33] Caring is both the prevention and the treatment for burnout. Only when engaged, can a nurse be a competent nurse, and only then can a nurse attain the level of job satisfaction that plays a part in growth of spirit. Furthermore, active engagement turns into a source of pride not only for the individual nurse, but for the profession of nursing as well.

In this last part of the book, I build upon the ways, already presented, to enter a patient's world of suffering in order to become a healing nurse. I will summarize and reinforce the information applying directly to practice that you have already learned. Then I will show you some specific interventions that will increase your capacity to care about yourself and others. While caring comes from the heart, armed with therapeutic techniques that I have taught for many years, you will learn how to handle difficult situations in ways that are affirming and restorative instead of discounting and distancing. Finally, I will discuss briefly the health care environment in which the patient and the nurse derive emergent support for caring.

Chapter XI

Avoiding Pitfalls and Burnout: Learning the Wisdom of Caring

The late psychiatrist, Viktor Frankl[34] noted that we grow as humans by allowing suffering into our experience. If this is really the case, healing nurses have the potential to be among the strongest of all people on earth. We are surrounded by suffering and we suffer as a result. Younger[35] has pointed out that the alienation experienced by people suffering in illness can be bridged by a wise person, a person who does not flee into superficiality when confronted by pain, and by persons who accept their *shadow side*, the negative and dark side that we all possess, but often try to hide by projecting the faults that lie in our own shadows onto others.

But how do nurses become wise instead of distressed when enclosed into a circle of suffering human kind, a world of untold injury that they cannot fix? Wisdom surfaces when involvement overrides the reaction to create distance from patients in order to avoid pain. We cannot restore a dead child or grandmother nor can we repair many disease processes. We cannot take away an abuse victim's pain. Many physical symptoms defy the most determined interventions. Feelings of failure become the enemy that assaults our self-esteem and grinds us into a self-protective mode aimed at personal survival, making us prime candidates to become the nurse who leaves nursing to sell real estate. Clearly the way that we face up to the suffering we encounter, including our own, can lead to highest wisdom or lowest forms of despair. The ever present dilemma for healing nurses is burnout versus a sense of reformed identity as competent human beings and professionals.

You cannot give what you do not have, so my first bit of advice is to find ways that you will use frequently to fortify yourself for wading around in the soggy trough of pain and fear that accompany disease. We might take stock of social and personal habits that drain our energy and create illness.[36, 37] It is not especially difficult to discover and learn some of the many self-examination techniques that can help make us wise. But in my experience, nurses tend to be givers, not takers. We cannot justify the time it takes to heal ourselves. In thoughtful group discussions with your peers, I suggest that you take on, as a critical issue, ways that each of you can begin to take back some of your own energy so that you will be replenished for the activities required of a healing nurse.

For a compact reference, I will summarize here in capsule form, the practical and philosophical advice I have given you throughout the book on how to practice healing nursing. I suggest that for a while, you keep your book open to these pages and review daily how you are doing in all these areas.

We learned:

- The importance of keeping up with scientific findings. One of the most caring things a nurse can do is to be competent by selecting interventions that are based upon evidence;
- How to be an ethical person and an ethical nurse by examining honestly our own values when dilemmas arise, facing up to our moral responsibilities to those who depend upon us, and accepting the accountability to guard a patient's right to self-determination;
- How we can arrive at a clearer understanding of our responsibility to patients by allowing into our consciousness the art of nursing and artistic and personal ways of illuminating what is good and right;
- How we can avoid the role entrapment barrier of being above the patient, instead assuming the character of an ordinary person whose whole self is engaged with the whole self of the patient;
- How to use the components of a caring relationship, such as forming a listening presence, supporting a patient's will to live and fight, intervening in fear of abandonment and neglect, and learning how to love the unlovable through empathy;
- And finally, we learned the importance of a very difficult role that must be enacted in a supportive environment –patient advocacy.

From these lessons we can pull out the following approaches that we can use with success in patient relationships and indeed in all relationships. Healing nursing requires that these skills and attitudes be formulated first in the nurse' mind and then honed in practice:

- Concentrated attention to the patient's condition and needs;
- An attitude of honesty, openness, and integrity;
- An ability to give encouragement;
- The courage to be creative and unrelenting in looking for solutions;
- The willingness to engage in compassionate and empathic communication.

Furthermore, we learned that healing nurses accept the responsibility to assist patients in attaining the resources and mind-set for healing, including helping patients to identify physical and emotional strengths needed to surmount the physical challenges that illness has set before them. Since it is often the case that we overlook the unique reasons that patients may have for regaining health, helping patients identify their own reasons for getting well will set all efforts for recovery in a positive direction. Like all advice in this book, healing practices can best be identified and carried out when they are reinforced within a group of peers where each has a commitment to the health of all.

Discussion and Exercises

1. What do you think is going through the minds of the nurses who create more suffering for patients or do not choose to alleviate the conditions of suffering? Is there a social, spiritual, or psychological explanation that you would put forth to explain how nurses can participate in causing suffering? Then, be honest with yourself and identify when you have felt the same way -when you may have passed up opportunities to be the best nurse you can be for a patient.

2. Devote part of your time in your discussion groups to attend to the self-care needs of all members of the group. Additionally, come up with some activities that could enhance your emotional and physical ability to care. Among these ways of healing might be ways to improve health practices, energetic practices, such as yoga and Tai Chi, and spiritual practices like meditation, prayer, and relaxation.

3. Discuss ways to establish the meaning of an illness experience for a patient?

4. Draw on an actual patient example to devise ways of improving care using the approaches given in this chapter.

Chapter XII

Nurse Healing Through Therapeutic Techniques

In this chapter I will present intervention techniques synthesized from the myriad of material published in nursing, psychology, communication, and other fields. I have honed these approaches over the years to my own specifications in order to assist nurses who are not specialists in mental health to improve their efforts at counseling. They require practice, so as you read through each part of this chapter, think how you might apply them to your work, then begin to try them out in your professional and personal life to effect better communication. I have found that role-playing, either with an audience or televised feedback, is an excellent way to learn more about your personal way of conveying caring through interpersonal techniques.

Showing caring through non-verbal communication

A healing interaction begins with nonverbal communication. Very little of our impression of each other is informed by what is said in words. Others attend to what we say with our bodies, facial expressions, and eyes. For example, I am very taken with the way that pharmaceutical companies advertise drugs on television. They are required by law to read the side-effects as part of the advertisement, but this lengthy accounting of potential danger is always accompanied by pictures of people smiling or engaging in peaceful or enjoyable activities. The eye and ear are drawn to the pictures, not the words.

A healing interaction starts **with looking patients in the eye** when you talk with them, maintaining eye contact for as much of the time as you can while performing other tasks. Even when you are taking a history, try to look up from your notes to the patient as often as you can. But take care when caring for patients from cultures that avoid direct eye contact. Minarik, an accomplished psychiatric nurse clinical specialist, suggested that for some Native Americans, for example, eye contact would be most inappropriate[38]. She relayed a story about a Native American staff member who, when she made direct eye contact, turned slightly to avoid her gaze. Only when she averted her gaze would he look back at her. He explained to her that direct eye contact is an affront in his culture. If your patient refuses to look back into your eyes, try turning your head a bit to the side during the conversation and see if that helps to relax him or her.

You will create a caring and listening presence by an **open body stance** –arms and legs uncrossed. **Leaning in toward patients** when listening, conveys an interest and careful hearing out of their ideas. Sit or stand at a **comfortable distance** from people. Use your own sense of distance as a guide, and then if you note that the patient is trying to create more distance, move back; or if the patient tries to move closer, you may decrease your distance.

All of your body needs to convey that what the patient is saying is the most important thing you have ever heard in your life. Body language is accompanied by **appropriate facial expressions** of concern or humor. **Attending to your voice** –lowering its pitch, tone, and volume, will help your words get across the caring and empathy you are trying to express. Patients, like all people, take in all non-verbal signs of interest in evaluating a nurse's caring.

You can practice these non-verbal techniques everywhere you go: with patients; at the line in the grocery store or the post office; in family gatherings with your spouse or children; while speaking to your supervisor or your team members; when withdrawing money at the bank; before the mirror in your bathroom; and in countless other situations. In examining your personal and professional relationships, you may find that you have fallen into communication patterns with coworkers, family members, and friends that have become so routine that they are lacking in overt manifestations of caring. Pick a date that you will concentrate on showing an interest in these important others by using non-verbal techniques of caring. The miracle is that they start out as techniques, but when used, they evoke such a positive response and deepening of the relationship that what was once a technique simply becomes a way of relating with awareness and interest to everyone.

Responding to nonverbal and verbal communication
Similarly, we need to attend to the clues of non-verbal communication coming from patients. When talking with patients

and their family members who are in crisis, making crucial decisions, or dealing with a fearful situation, it is always appropriate to use your observations about non-verbal communication. You can note changes in voice pitch or intensity, or changes in posture that indicate closing up, such as hugging arms to the body, head down, or tight facial expression. Your response should never be in an accusatory tone of "You are standing on my foot!", or a lecturing attitude of "You are not trying hard enough." Instead it is to be conveyed in a soft, non-judgmental manner that indicates your interest and concern for going deeper than the superficial verbalization that we often get from patients who do not trust that we will care enough to listen. The formula for intervention is: state what you feel, say what you observed, and then invite a response, as in the following paragraph:

> "When you mentioned what your clinician told you about the findings of your scans and lab work, I **felt** a wave of apprehension and **experienced** a bit of your pushing me away. I **heard** your voice become worried and **saw** your body looking tense. I wonder if you could **say more about how you are feeling** about what is happening to you."

The following principles apply to all feedback that you give a patient:

- Make sure your feedback or questions are not judgmental or threatening.
- Never challenge the patient's view of reality. Just try to understand it.
- Use your physical presence, along with appropriate touch, to communicate empathy and caring.
- Use verbal and non-verbal listening approaches to get the whole story from the patient before you try to intervene.

Preparing for tense clinical situations
When entering a treatment room or other patient area in which you feel you may encounter conflict or extreme anxiety, you can start being therapeutic from the first minute you walk into the door by paying attention to the following hints:

- Stop at the door for a few seconds and listen carefully to orient yourself to the tone of what is happening. Take a deep breath then exhale slowly while you let your whole mind and body relax;

- Develop a personal mantra to say to yourself that focuses your mind on the purpose for your presence. Mine is, "I am here to give my best;"
- Anticipate and image a positive response to your presence;
- Open your body by relaxing your arms to your side;
- When you speak, lower the pitch of your voice.
- Maintain eye contact with whomever you speak.
- Maintain a pleasant or neutral facial expression.

Focusing on experiences and solutions, not problems

Mitchell, a clinical specialist practicing in Toronto, writes that she became aware that she was doing patients a disservice because she was focusing on their problems instead of their experiences.[39] Once she began offering herself in true presence, she no longer forced her own interpretations on the situation in the form of her diagnoses and judgments. Mitchell noted that while some universal patterns, such as stages of grief or stages of death might be generally informative, all meaning evolves from the patient's world and the patient's experience.

Believing this strongly, I always assume that the solution for any problem lies in the patient's unique strengths and that we will uncover that strength by listening to the patient's account of the problem or issue. When trying to do problem solving, the questions that we ask to unearth medical and psychological weakness or problems simply reinforce the patient's helplessness. To implement these principles, you can employ some of the tenets of solution-focused therapy,[40, 41] a form of brief therapy that has been used by professional psychiatric practitioners, including nurses, that delineates techniques and principles that apply to any situation encountered by a nurse.

Principles of solution-focused communication

- We must give up our presumptions about what the person is like or what the problem is based on a patient's diagnosis or disability.
- The material for solving the problem lies within the patient. The patient is the expert.
- A change in one part of the system affects the whole system. As a result, small changes tend to lead to big changes.
- The emphasis is on the future, not the past. So we do not need to know the cause to find the solution.

Solution-focused therapy does not take a great deal of time. In using solution-focused methods with a great many students and workshop participants, I have discovered that this method, which seems so ridiculously simple, results in the most incredible outcomes. In my workshops and classes, I put students in pairs, and ask them to share with each other an unwanted pattern or problem that they want to solve. Then they go through the steps of solution-focused therapy with each other. The enthusiasm at the end is hard to believe, and in subsequent evaluations, it is always mentioned as the most important thing they learned. Follow the exercises at the end of the chapter so that you can start your learning by seeing how effective the method is in dealing with solutions to your own unwanted patterns.

Techniques of solution-focused therapy
1. Establish clear goals
It is important to know how the person with the problem will know when the problem has been solved. What will they be doing and feeling? Ask them to describe in detail what a successful outcome will look like. Have the patient describe it so clearly that you could draw a picture of it. Ask them to tell you what will they be doing when the problem is solved? When early signs of improvement occur, the patient should be reminded to take note of this instead of dismissing it. For example, if an acutely ill patient wants to be able to be well enough to walk his daughter down the aisle at her wedding 6 months hence, then being able to walk to the bathroom with help is an early sign that should be noted and cheered. Other early signs concern possible changes in this man's personal health patterns, such as faithfulness to good medical regimes, exercise to the limit of his ability, attention to sound nutrition, and practice of any lifestyle choices that will eventually result in a healthier body.

2. Focus on strengths
Ask patients to describe a time in detail when they have successfully solved a problem in the past. This will not only give clues to their best ways of problem-solving, but will also encourage current efforts at problem-solving when they realize that indeed they have always had the ability to affect a solution. It is also helpful to ask the patient to remember a time when he/she did not have the problem, and to describe what things were like then. This description will set the

mind toward healthy aspects of the life and it also will contain clues to the solution. I like to encourage patients to talk about their strengths, their favorite activities, and what matters the most to them because I will often see a solution to the problem in this description. When somebody is ill, they are never asked about strength or what they enjoy or are good at doing. Instead, almost all dialogue concerns problems and disease.

For example, a patient of John Edwards,[42] one of my students at the University of Texas, was furious at her husband because he did not get to the hospital, which was far from their farm, in time to see her off to surgery. Her recovery and rehabilitation were severely retarded because she seemed to have given up. All she could think about was her fuming anger at her undependable husband, crying, "I could have died on the table." Instead of focusing on the anger or saying the usual sugary phrases that would placate her, Mr. Edwards changed the subject entirely and asked her what she would be doing at home when she got well. The patient became animated when talking about the farm and the everyday jobs that had always been such a valued part of her life on the farm. Building upon this, Mr. Edwards asked her to make a list of all the activities that needed doing when she got well, and who would do them, her or her husband. While completing this task, she became excited about returning to her work, and she began to cooperate with the staff on her rehabilitation. Her resentment faded out entirely, and her husband was finally allowed to explain to her that his car broke down on the way to the hospital. Mr. Edwards wrote,

> When I visited her for the last time in the hospital, she was smiling and confident about her plans for recovery and was talking in easy conversation with her husband. The sense of fulfillment which washed over me at this point is beyond description. While I was not able to solve her problems, I was able to assist her in providing a structure or meaning to her recovery that eventually led to renewed strengths and bonding between her and her husband.

3. Reframe
Offer another explanation of the problem that fits the facts but makes the problem more solvable. When counseling patients who have a life threatening illness, I reframe fear of dying as a normal

coping mechanism, a strong way that nature has of protecting us from harm when we sense that our bodies are in danger. I then turn the attention to all the things that this normal stress reaction may be teaching us or directing us to do. An unsolvable grief reaction can be reframed as a sadness that shows that the person has cared deeply. Starting on a rigorous diet and exercise program for a hard-working person who is too busy doing things for other people, can be reframed as an opportunity to do something for oneself.

4. Pattern intervention

We all carry out the activities of our day using long established patterns, some of which we learned as children. For example, when dressing I always put on my right shoe before I put on my left shoe. If you were repeatedly given an after-school snack by your mother, this may now continue in the form of always grabbing something to eat when returning home. Such automatic behaviors can be helpful in circumventing the need to make many small decisions all day, but some may retard attempts to change health habits as adults. In the case of a snack that is contributing to weight gain, avoiding walking through kitchen when returning home can disrupt a portion of the negative pattern. Putting on leisure clothes and going out to work in the garden for a few minutes before having the snack will also interrupt this eating pattern eventually, and is a way of substituting positive patterns to replace negative patterns. One simple exercise I give to patients who do this is to change their clothes first, then stop just before entering the kitchen and engage in 5 minutes of deep breathing and stretching exercises.

First, get a description of the pattern from the person. If the person cannot sleep, and assuming this is not a physical or chemical problem, suggest one change in the going to bed ritual - stay up an hour later, for example, or read a chapter in a book instead of watching a movie on TV. Remember that one of the principles of pattern intervention is that when one part of the system changes, the entire system has to adjust, so it does not matter so much what you suggest in the going to bed ritual as long as it disrupts the usual pattern.

One of my recent patients was a man who after his heart attack felt he did not have time to do the prescribed exercise. I could see that he did not have time because his patterns from arising to bedtime were sedentary and fixed to not allow time for this activity —yet on observation, there were many instances during the day when he could have exercised. I asked him what time of day he would feel the most like exercising. Since it was early evening, just before dinner, I assisted him to change his pattern by changing what he did just before dinner. I asked him to go outside, walk one block, and return to the house. Remember when changing a pattern, you only need to change a small part of it. Turn calls this tossing in a monkey wrench.[43] So, although the eventual goal for this patient was to exercise for 30 minutes four times a week, walking one block was a start on that goal that disrupted the sedentary pattern enough to allow inclusion of a new health behavior in the day. In fact, what happened is that he began to walk for 10 to 15 minutes before dinner, and then after dinner he started to walk with his wife for a period of at least 30 minutes. They ended up back at their own block where they talked and gossiped with neighbors, disrupting a pattern of going back to their den, and sitting down to watch TV all evening while eating snacks of popcorn and chips.

Discussion and Exercises

1. Develop a scenario of an actual patient you have cared for who was in a health crisis. Practice using the non-verbal techniques of concerned listening: open body stance, leaning toward the patient, eye contact, and appropriate facial expression for the situation. Give each other direct feedback and allow repeating of the role playing, if necessary. If possible, videotape these sessions to give direct feedback to the person playing the nurse. Seeing yourself on tape will be a surprise to most nurses, who will find that they have much more empathetic gestures than they may have given themselves credit for.

2. Locate in your own life one pattern or a habit that you would like to change. With a partner, go through the techniques of Solution-focused therapy to change that pattern. After you make a plan, carry it out. Reverse roles and play the therapist for your partner.

Chapter XIII

The Healing Environment

> *No man is an island, entire of it self; ...*
> *Any man's death diminishes me, because I am involved in mankind; And*
> *therefore never send to know for whom the bell tolls; It tolls for thee.* [44]
> *- John Donne*

John Donne's famous poem puts into words the universal exigency for connection to the whole –the consolation of being able to dip into vast environmental resources for support, recognition, encouragement, and most fundamentally, to define who we are as human beings. Moreover, there is no room in a service profession for isolated egos –grasping and competing; denying and judging. Nurses began to form their nursing identity the first day of nursing school, heeding the examples and the remarks of teachers and peers. Typically, few experiences in your school of nursing were designed to promote nurse cohesion and to assist you in reaching out to peers and mentors for courage and confirmation when you were trying to grasp the meaning of your patient's and your own distress. As such, they did not prepare you for ways you will need to attain support for your practice throughout a lifetime.

It is an easy task for a writer to use the pages of this chapter to rail about the conditions that now prevail in nursing organizations, a state of affairs that has cast such a pall on the advancement of good patient care. Such criticisms are ensconced into the ambient nursing culture and burned onto our foreheads. Academicians and clinicians wonder how nursing can move ahead on developing its art and science when administrators have to worry day and night about the sheer number of bodies available to carry out care –from which country can they entice an immigrant, from whom can they steal another nurse. This subject is on the minds of everyone in nursing from the beginning student to the President of the American Nurses' Association.

It is true that there is a severe shortage. We need more nurses than ever before to fill the huge number of expanding, even exciting roles that have been created in all aspects of the health care system. We also need more nurses to operate and oversee complex machines and drug regimes. Increasingly an individual nurse can monitor many fewer patients, as unit acuity levels rise to unheard of heights. Strained to the limit, nurses are upset about multiple unsupportive conditions under which they work that drive more promising practitioners away from the field every year.

In a scathing indictment of nurse to nurse support, students in the first year of school hear the atrocious phrase, "Nurses eat their young." And many of them I have talked with believe it and feel that it will affect them now and in the future. In a letter to the editor in the *American Nurse*, a member of the Florida Nurses' Association, Sean E. McMicken, addressed this lack of support of nurses by nurses.[45] Then he goes on to say,

> If Dr. Unknown makes a mistake or social *faux pas*, we immediately rally behind him with encouragement and gentle remediation. Almost always he admits within our secret circle that he should have done or said something different. He knows his confession and learning are safe with us... Nursing must create an environment of support, starting in our academic centers and develop mentors who care.

Helpless to respond to such an array of environmental problems, nurses try to find ways of just getting through the rather long hours that have now become a shift. Even in an outpatient practice, nurses must see upwards of 20 patients with complex problems per day, which keeps their exhausted noses firmly affixed to the grindstone. But there are rational approaches to ameliorating a non-supportive practice environment that limits the work week to endless problems, one after the next, with no opportunity for collaboration and encouragement. One can be found in the book by nurse advocate, speaker, and writer, Peggy Chinn.[46] She writes about using ongoing group process to find means of reflecting our words in actions -connecting what we know with what we do. In her book, *Peace and Power*, which can be used by nurses as a manual, she teaches practical processes that build upon principles of unity and that can be implemented in large and small groups. Group unity starts with clarifying a group's purpose, and sharing our beliefs, values, and expectations of each other. In nursing, such processes must be enacted in ongoing, face-to-face groups that are structured for the purpose of learning more about the vast complexity of what appears to be such a simple skill –the art of nursing.

Sherman[47] has identified the factors that cause stress in nurses, in a list that includes personal, professional and system variables. She suggests that nurses become advocates for themselves and each other and that they turn their attention to self care activities, including attention to their own health and energy level. She reasons that if nurses recognize early when they are burning out, they can take steps to renew themselves for the demands of the workplace. Her all too brief attempt at suggesting systems interventions concern asking nurses to join their specialty association in order to have more knowledge about care and discussing professional roles and ethics among themselves.

So although the problem is enormous, there are emerging solutions, waiting to be employed by anyone who has the vitality and the courage to confront apathy and indifference by refusing to give in. As I wrote this book, I pictured you, the readers, as healing nurses, going head to head with the concepts and the suggestions that I have outlined, while fashioning a broader appreciation of your rights and responsibility as a nurse. I wanted you fortified with the knowledge whereby nursing derives its reason for being. I wanted to picture you as an ethical and thoughtful nurse who forms care by embracing both science and art. I wanted you to come to your practice fully armed with the wisdom you would need to solve the most perplexing problems of care. Yet, I am fully aware that an encouraging group is a fundamental prerequisite for enacting much of what I have outlined –a group that will contribute to your growing knowledge and help you to shape an alliance for turning your work environment into a thriving atmosphere for patient and employee health.

For example, three of my advanced RN students, who were taking my master's level course, called *Caring and Helping in Nursing*, and were becoming true healing nurses, worked together in an emergency room. When doing the class exercises similar to those at the end of each chapter of this book, they begin to formulate in reality how they could make a difference in their real life clinical setting. In the beginning the others on the ER staff were rather puzzled at the unfamiliar practices of these nurses, as they took a few minutes here and there to be in presence with patients, or took measures to calm troubled staff and patient situations. Initially the staff would explain to observers, "Don't mind them, they are taking a course at the university called, *Caring and Helping in Nursing*." At length, the atmosphere in the ER began to change and some staff changed their approaches a bit when these students were on duty. Finally, the students reported that they began to have more team meetings with all the staff that were professionally geared to improvement of patient care.

Following the advice and using the information in this book can open doors for a renewal of nursing that will help us attain hoped-for advancement in our profession. Success lies first in studying the fundamentals of your professional practice. And too, remember the lesson that we all have different talents to contribute to care. Similarly, we all have special talents we bring to system change. By working in a team that is utilizing nursing knowledge and devoted to improving care and working conditions, each can contribute in her or his own way to the welfare of all.

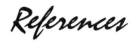

References

1. Quinn, J. (1996). *Therapeutic touch: Healing through energy fields.* NY: National League for Nursing and University of Colorado Center for Human Caring.

2. Helminiak, DA. (1996). *The human core of spirituality: Mind as psyche and spirit.* New York: SUNY Press.

3. Hall, BA. & Allan, JD (1994). Self in Relation: A prolegomenon for holistic nursing. *Nursing Outlook, 15,* 110-116

4. Niedowaki, E. (Feb 9, 2002). The Artful doctor. *Baltimore Sun,* page 8a.

5. *Nursing's social policy statement (2nd Ed.).* (2003). Washington DC: American Nurses Association.

6. Fawcett, J. (1989). *Analysis and evaluation of conceptual models of nursing (2nd ed.).* Philadelphia: Davis.

7. Taylor, BJ. (1992). Caring: Being manifested as ordinariness in nursing. In DA Gout (ed), *The presence of caring in nursing.* 182-200. New York: NLN.

8. Carper, BA. (1978). Fundamental patterns of knowing in nursing. *Advances in Nursing Science,* 113-23.

9. Chinn, PL. & Kramer, MK. (2003) *Integrated knowledge development. (6th ed.).* St. Louis: CV Mosby.

10. Godwin, G. (1994). *The good husband.* New York: Ballantine Books.

11. Barnsteiner, J. & Prevost, S. (2002). How to implement evidence-based practice: Some tried and true pointers. *Reflections on Nursing Leadership. 28.* 18-21.

12. White, J. (1995). Patterns of knowing: Review, critique, and update. *Advances in Nursing Science, 17,* 73-86.

13. Callahan, D. (1994). *Bioethics: Private choice and common good.* Hastings Center Report, May-June, 87.

14. Parker, RS. (1990). Nurses' stories: The search for a relational ethic of care. *Advances in Nursing Science, 13,* 31-40.

15. Aristotle. (1962). *Nicomachean ethics:* Translated with and introduction and notes by Martin Ostwald. New York: Macmillan/The library of the liberal arts.

16. Schecter, S. (1990). *The AIDS notebooks.* New York: SUNY Press.

17. *Selected Poems of Anne Sexton.* (1988). Boston: Mariner.

18. Frost, R. (1962). Poem read at the inauguration of John F Kennedy.

19. Noddings, N. (1984). *Caring: A feminine approach to ethics & moral education.* Berkeley: University of California Press.

20. Dass, R. & Gorman, P. (1987). *How Can I help?* New York: Alfred A. Knopf.

21. Hall, BA. (1996). The psychiatric model: A critical analysis of its undermining effects on nursing in chronic mental illness. *Advances in Nursing Science, 18,* 16-26.

22. Mitchell, G. (1990). Struggling in change: From the traditional approach to Parse's theory-based practice. *Nursing Science Quarterly, Winter,* 170-176.

23. Kennedy, G. (1995). Personal Story.

24. Montgomery CL. (1993). *Healing through communication.* Newbury Park: Sage.

25. Hall, B.A. (1993). Time in Nursing: Reflections of an aging nurse-radical. *Nursing Outlook, 41,* 250-252.

26. Budgen, C. (1988). Patients' and families' perceptions of quality of nursing care: Exploring the association between process and outcome. Unpublished PhD Dissertation. Austin: University of Texas.

27. Middlebrook, DW. (1991). *Anne Sexton: A biography.* New York: Vintage Books.

28. Gadow, S. (1990) Nursing: The Advocacy Covenant: Care as clinical subjectivity. *Images and Ideals: Opening dialogue with the humanities.* Kansas City: The American Academy of Nursing.

29. Sheridan, SL. Harris, RP. Woolf, SH. (2004). Shared decision making about screening and chemoprevention. *American Journal of Preventive Medicine: 26,* 56-66.

30. Porter-O'Grady, T. & Malloch, K. (2002). *Quantum Leadership: A textbook of new leadership.* Aspen: Gaithersburg, MD.

31. Falk-Rafael, AR. (2001). Empowerment as a process of evolving consciousness: A model of empowered caring, *Advances in Nursing Science, 24,* 1-16.

32. Stark, M. (1979). *Nightingale's Cassandra.* Westbury, Con: Feminist Press.

33. Benner, P. (1984). *From novice to expert.* Menlo Park CA: Addison-Wesley.

34. Frankl, V. (1959). *Man's search for meaning.* New York: Simon & Shuster.

35. Younger, JB. (1995). The alienation of the sufferer. *Advances in Nursing Science, 17,* 53-73.

36. McGinnis, M., Foege, WH. (1993). Actual causes of death in the United States. *Journal of the American Medical Association 270,* 2207-2212.

37. Hall, BA. (2003). *Surviving and thriving after a life threatening diagnosis.* Bloomington, ID: 1st Books Library.

38. Minarik, PA. (2005). Personal Communication.

39. Mitchell, GJ. (1990). Struggling in change: From the traditional approach to Parse's theory based practice. *Nursing Science Quarterly, Winter,* 170-176.

40. Walter, JL., Peller, JE. (1992). *Becoming solution-focused in brief therapy.* New York: Brunner-Mazel.

41. Webster, DC., Vaughn, K., & Martinez, R. (1992). Introducing solution-focused approaches to staff in inpatient psychiatric settings. *Archives of Psychiatric Nursing,* 254-260.

42. Edwards, JR (1997). Solution-oriented therapy under the umbrella of meaning and existential advocacy. Unpublished class assignment.

43. Turn, LK. (1992). Solution-oriented therapy and Rogerian science: An integrated approach. Archives of Psychiatric Nursing, 6, 83-89.

44. Donne, J. (1624). *Devotions upon emergent occasions*.

45. McMicken, SE. (2004). Letter to the editor: Support for Nurses Needed. *American Nurse, January/February*.

46. Chinn, PL. (2004). Peace *and Power: Creative Leadership for Building Community, (6th ed.)*. New York: Jones and Bartlett.

47. Sherman, DW. (2004). Nurses' stress and burnout. *American Journal of Nursing, 104*, 8-56.